Nurse Practitioners:
Developing the Role in H̶o̶s̶p̶i̶t̶a̶l̶ ̶S̶e̶t̶t̶i̶n̶g̶s̶

Commissioning Editor: Mary Seager
Development Editor: Caroline Savage
Production Controller: Anthony Read
Desk Editor: Deena Burgess
Cover Designer: Alan Studholme

Nurse Practitioners: Developing the Role in Hospital Settings

Edited by

Shirley Reveley, Phd, MA, BA, RGN, RM, RHV, DipN (London), CertEd,
Head of Department of Nursing Studies, St Martin's College,
Lancaster & Carlisle, UK

Mike Walsh, PhD, BA (Hons), RGN, PGCE, DipN (London),
Reader in Nursing, St Martin's College, Lancaster & Carlisle, UK

Alison Crumbie, MSN, BSc, RGN, DipNP, Dip App ScN, PGCE,
Nurse Practitioner, St Martin's College, Lancaster & Carlisle, UK

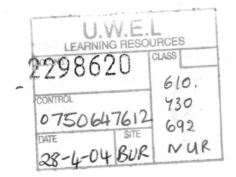
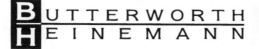

BUTTERWORTH
HEINEMANN

OXFORD   AUCKLAND   BOSTON   JOHANNESBURG   MELBOURNE   NEW DELHI

Butterworth-Heinemann
Linacre House, Jordan Hill, Oxford OX2 8DP
225 Wildwood Avenue, Woburn, MA 01801-2041
A division of Reed Educational and Professional Publishing Ltd

℞ A member of the Reed Elsevier plc group

First published 2001

British Library Cataloguing in Publication Data
Nurse practitioners: developing the role in hospital settings
  1. Nurse practitioners
  I. Reveley, Shirley   II. Walsh, Mike, 1949–   III. Crumbie, Alison
  610.7'30692

ISBN 0 7506 4761 2

Typeset by E & M Graphics, Midsomer Norton, Bath

Printed and bound in Great Britain by MPG Books Ltd, Bodmin, Cornwall

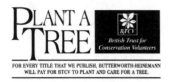

CONTENTS

CONTRIBUTORS

Chris Batten, BA, Grad.Dip.Out.Ed, Grad.Dip.Mktg Mgt, MSc
Business Development Manager, Wilmslow, Manchester. Management Consultant (Organisation Development, Marketing and Leadership); Executive member of the Board of Directors for the International Association for Experimental Education.

Lesley Carruthers, BSc (Hons)
Clinical Nurse Practitioner, Orthopaedic Department, West Cumberland Hospital, Cumbria.

Alison Crumbie, MSN, BSc, RGN, DipNP, Dip App ScN, PGCE
Nurse Practitioner and Senior Lecturer at St Martin's College, Lancaster. Course leader for the nurse practitioner syllabus at St Martin's and a founding member of the Northern Nurse Practitioner Association.

Kathy Haigh, BSc (Hons), RCNI
Nurse Practitioner, General Surgery at Blackpool Victoria NHS Trust.

Shirley Reveley, PhD, MA, BA, RGN, RM, RHV, DipN (London), CertEd
Principal Lecturer, St Martin's College, Carlisle. Responsible for setting up a nurse practitioner programme in Carlisle and Lancaster in association with the RCN Institute. Research interests include evaluating the nurse practitioner role.

Fiona Smart, MA Bed (Hons), RGN, RSCN, DipN, RNT
Programme Manager, Child Health and Children's Nursing, St Martin's College, Carlisle.

Mike Walsh, PhD, BA (Hons), RGN, PGCE, DipN (London)
Reader in Nursing, St Martin's College, Carlisle. Background in A&E nursing, research and practice development. Well known for a range of books and journal articles on both clinical and professional issues.

PREFACE

The role of the nurse practitioner in the United Kingdom has come of age. From its beginnings in primary care in the early 1980s, the nurse practitioners movement has developed rapidly and nurse practitioners can now be found in every area of health care. Despite the obvious success of the nurse practitioner role there are still no minimum standards of practice and education laid in statute, and the United Kingdom Central Council for Nursing, Midwifery and Health Visiting (UKCC) has failed to clarify, or even acknowledge, this important new role.

This book celebrates nurse practitioners. It is written by proponents of the role and the three editors are steeped in researching the role of the nurse practitioner and educating nurse practitioners in both primary care and hospital settings. The book is intended for nurse practitioner students, practising nurse practitioners, educationalists, managers and health professionals who come into contact with nurse practitioners in the course of their work. It is intended to deepen understanding of the role and set nurse practitioners' work in the context of modern health care delivery. Although written with hospital-based nurse practitioners in mind, the book is appropriate reading for nurse practitioners in every clinical setting because it covers such important generic issues as marketing, educating and evaluating the role.

The book is structured in three parts: Part 1 provides an overview of the development of the nurse practitioner role and sets it into context of recent policy initiatives such as the National Health Service Plan. The thorny issue of nurse practitioners and clinical nurse specialist roles is picked up, and the vexed question of levels of nursing practice is explored. Because the roles of nurse practitioners and junior doctors in hospital are so closely entwined, Chapter 4 examines the relationships of nurse practitioners and doctors to one another and to patients, and raises the issue of jurisdiction over patient care.

Part 2 takes a practical focus. Two nurse practitioners talk about their work. Although they work in different hospitals many miles apart, and do not know each other, there are many similarities in their *modus operandi*. In Chapter 5, a surgical nurse practitioner describes her particular journey from experienced nurse to nurse practitioner. The stages of development she went through and her experiences in attempting to develop the role on the unit are, in our experience, very common in nurses undergoing role transition.

In Chapter 6, a nurse practitioner in an orthopaedic unit describes how she introduced a nurse practitioner-led pre-operative assessment clinic into the hospital. The perceptions of some health professionals towards her work are discussed, and some of the barriers she had to overcome are described. These two chapters are accompanied by commentaries on the role; the first by a consultant anaesthetist and the second by a patient.

In Chapter 7 a new nurse practitioner role is described, that of the paediatric nurse practitioner. This role is in the early stages of development in the UK, and Fiona Smart discusses plans and emerging issues. Chapter 8 is concerned with nurse practitioners at the interface of primary and secondary care; in the accident and emergency department, minor injuries unit, walk-in-centres and other innovative areas of practice.

Part 3 addresses the issues of education, marketing and evaluating the role of the nurse practitioner. These themes are common to nurse practitioners whatever the setting, and are vitally important to the successful implementation and development of the role.

We hope you enjoy reading this book and find it both enlightening and useful.

Shirley Reveley
Mike Walsh
Alison Crumbie

PART 1

The political and professional context of the nurse practitioner movement in the UK

THE NURSE PRACTITIONER AND HOSPITAL-BASED CARE; SETTING THE SCENE

Mike Walsh

Every bristling shaft of pride
Church or nation
Team or tribe,
Every notion we subscribe to
Is just a borderline.
Borderline by Joni Mitchell (1994)

Introduction

Introducing and developing the nurse practitioner role in hospital settings is all about borderlines. Joni Mitchell's lyrics are very apposite, as hospitals are populated by 'teams and tribes' called professions. It is not surprising that when one of those tribes attempts to expand its area of activity, bordering tribes become anxious or even hostile, and this may potentially result in what our North American colleagues call a turf war. Nurse practitioners are attempting to develop nursing practice to a new level and are doing so for the benefit of patients, not for their own kudos. This development is occurring at the borders of nursing and medicine, and there are those on both sides of that border who feel threatened by this movement. As a result, the unwary nurse can find herself impaled upon 'bristling shafts of pride'. In the past, some statutory bodies have made little constructive contribution to the nurse practitioner debate and it would do them well to pay heed to Francis Bacon's observation that 'Silence is the virtue of fools'.

As we write this book, the government has just launched its NHS Plan to reform and modernize the NHS. We believe nurse practitioners can play a major part in the fulfilment of that plan, and this book is an attempt to show how the role can be implemented in our hospitals. The nurse practitioner is a new and challenging concept, especially in secondary care where, over the decades, professional boundaries have become etched into the very

fabric of our hospitals. As the immediate Past President of the Emergency Nurses Association of the USA, Jean Proehl, observed: 'The old ways of doing things just get you the old results' (Proehl, 2000). If we want new and better results for the NHS, we have to find new ways of working. The nurse practitioner concept offers one such route both in primary and hospital care settings, but it does mean we have to redraw some of the old borderlines as they will only hinder progress as they are at present.

The historical development of the nurse practitioner role

The nurse practitioner role is not new. It originated in the USA during the 1960s, at first as a means to help improve health care for rural populations, especially children. The two early pioneers were Loretta Ford (a nurse) and Henry Silver (a doctor). The role therefore originated as a result of interdisciplinary co-operation between innovative and forward-looking doctors and nurses whose main concern was improving health care for patients. It very quickly became adopted across the USA, and university-based education for the role was rapidly developed. The three key principles were therefore established over 30 years ago, and remain as relevant today as they did then:

1. The role is primarily for the benefit of the patient
2. Inter-professional collaboration between medicine and nursing is essential
3. The nurse practitioner should have a university-based, graduate, educational preparation for the role.

These three principles are an absolutely essential underpinning for the hospital-based role as it develops in the new century. The prime reason for introducing the nurse practitioner role in hospitals has to be improving patient care; not making it easier to implement mandatory reductions in junior doctors' hours, possibly providing cheaper care, or because it sounds a trendy thing to be doing. This also means that it has to be possible to show subsequently that patient care has benefited from nurse practitioner introduction. The role cannot be effectively introduced unless there is goodwill and co-operation from all the other groups of staff involved, especially but not solely from medical staff. This has major implications for the strategies that have to be followed to introduce radical changes to what are, in many cases, century-old working practices.

The nurse practitioner must have education that is fit for purpose in order to be both effective and safe. This means that an Honours degree preparation is the minimum that is acceptable. Close links are necessary with higher education to ensure the correct amount of academic rigour is combined with practical experience to produce a course that is relevant to the needs of both patient and nurse practitioner. As doctors obtain their licence to practise with education at Honours degree level, we feel that nurse practitioners should have the same basic academic level of pre-paration. Master's level education should not be the minimum standard, but should be available to those nurse practitioners who wish to pursue their studies and research further.

The three key issues of rationale, inter-disciplinary collaboration and education have been introduced here because they are so important, and they will be explored in considerable depth in subsequent chapters.

The nurse practitioner role, supported by a strong university-based education programme, rapidly developed in the USA during the 1970s, and a major survey by Running *et al.* (2000) estimates there are now 60 000 nurse practitioners in the USA of whom 86 per cent are graduates at Bachelors or Masters level. The pioneering work of Barbara Stilwell brought the role to the UK in the 1980s, originally with a strong primary health care focus. However, as early pilot studies were demonstrating the feasibility of the primary health care nurse practitioner in the NHS, the role was beginning to find its way into North American hospitals, initially into the field of emergency care. The Emergency Room was expanding to become the Emergency Department in larger hospitals. It quickly became apparent that nurses with nurse practitioner skills could provide a fast-track service, allowing many patients with less serious conditions to be seen quickly by a nurse practitioner rather than endure a lengthy wait to see a physician. This however was only possible if the nurse practitioner could order radiographs and had prescriptive authority. These issues have been largely worked through in the USA but remain major problems in the NHS, not only for the nurse practitioner working in A&E, but also for nurse practi-tioners across the hospital sector. Once again we are back to the issue of borderlines and other professional groups (such as radio-graphers and pharmacists) opposing the expansion of nursing roles.

When the nurse practitioner movement began to develop in hospitals in the USA it found clinical nurse specialists were already a well-established group. Much debate has surrounded these two titles, but the trend has been for the roles to merge together under the banner of the advanced practice nurse. Running *et al.* (2000) reported that 17.8 per cent of nurse practitioners were classified as advanced practice nurses in their study, indicating the steady growth of the nurse practitioner role in hospital care in the USA. As with many things, we have tended to follow North American trends and developments in this field. Nurses working in A&E were the 'early adopters' of the nurse practitioner concept in British hospitals, and now the nurse practitioner is becoming widespread in our hospitals but under a somewhat confusing array of titles.

As there is no definition of the nurse practitioner role in the United Kingdom, there is no national educational standard or central record of nurses who are entitled to use the title of nurse practitioner. As we shall see in the next chapter, this has caused many problems for nurses and patients. It is illustrative of the confusion that nurses working in A&E have been keen to adopt the title of emergency nurse practitioner from their North American colleagues. The only problem is that many nurses using the emergency nurse practitioner title do not possess a degree-level nurse practitioner education and are not seeing patients who are emergencies, making the title a complete misnomer! We feel that the UKCC should recognize the nurse practitioner concept and adopt a title such as advanced practice nurse or something similar. The UKCC have withdrawn their original proposals for advanced and specialist practice contained in the launch of their PREP document in 1994 and have now proposed the Higher Level of Practice (HLP) as an alternative designation for advanced nursing practice. The HLP project is currently being piloted by the UKCC, and this will be explored further in Chapter 3.

The last decade witnessed the rapid expansion of the nurse practitioner movement in the UK, and the first course offered by a national body, the Royal College of Nursing Institute, was a Nurse Practitioner Diploma, which was quickly upgraded to Honours degree level. A series of Higher Education Institutions franchised the RCNI course, including St Martin's College, which is where the authors work and which has campuses in Lancaster and in Cumbria. We started offering the course in January 1995 and quickly began to attract applications from hospital-based students, with the result that, by 1998, approximately half our recruits were from the hospital sector. The demand for specialization has led to the original hospital route through the programme being replaced by three routes: paediatrics, A&E and acute hospital care. Within the UK we are now seeing the same debate taking place regarding the clinical nurse specialist or nurse practitioner role as has previously occurred in the USA.

Our basic position is that the nurse practitioner degree programme was originally developed around a set of core skills that the nurse practitioner could deploy in a primary health care setting. However the key skills of taking a medical history, carrying out a physical examination and utilizing diagnostic reasoning to build on a nursing assessment are equally valid and important in any clinical environment. The underpinning knowledge of pathophysiology and applied pharmacology is also just as valid whether the patient is in a local health centre, an A&E unit or the outpatients department of a district general hospital. There is therefore no reason why nurse practitioners cannot practise in a specialist area such as urology or orthopaedics,

provided that they are given guidance about how to apply the basic tool-kit of skills and knowledge acquired on the course to their clinical speciality. Many of the hospital-based students who are going through our BSc Nurse Practitioner course are clinical nurse specialists who are developing and expanding their role into a hospital advanced practice nurse. The debate about being a specialist or generalist is therefore meaningless, as a well-thought-through degree programme can equip students for either role.

The nurse practitioner role has therefore developed dramatically in a very short period in the UK and has come in from the community to the hospital setting via the A&E department. All this has happened largely in the space of a single decade, and without the support of the UKCC. It is ironic therefore to reflect upon the fact that none of this could have happened without the UKCC document *The Scope of Professional Practice* (UKCC, 1992). As Walsh has argued elsewhere, the UKCC let the genie out of the bottle with their *Scope* document and now do not seem to know what to do with it, having spent the last 9 years trying to push it back in (Walsh, 2000).

The Scope of Professional Practice represents a major landmark in the development of British nursing, and the UKCC should be congratulated on its production. This document freed nursing from the strait-jacket of the *Extended Role of the Nurse* circular (DHSS, 1977). This document was purely task-focused, and stated that a nurse may only undertake additional tasks if they were delegated by a doctor and deemed appropriate for nurses to carry out (without actually saying who would 'deem appropriate' whatever tasks were involved). Nursing was therefore very much cast in the subordinate role to medicine, as only doctors could decide how nurses would expand or extend their practice. This document also saw nursing purely in terms of tasks rather than as a whole activity whose purpose was to benefit the patient. As we seek to implement the nurse practitioner role in hospitals in a new century, we must be aware that the ghosts of task orientation and medical domination have not been fully laid by the *Scope of Professional Practice* document.

The *Extended Role of the Nurse* circular also led to nurses having to carry around certificates of competence for all the various tasks they were allowed to undertake. This led to many problems, the most common of which was that one hospital would not recognize another hospital's certificates whenever a nurse moved jobs. There was also an assumption that the person issuing the certificate was competent, an assumption which is questionable to say the least. Furthermore, although the nurse might have been competent when assessed, that was no guarantee that this was still the case 2 years later.

The *Scope of Professional Practice* document cancelled the 1977 DHSS *Extended Role of the Nurse* circular and replaced it with a set of guidelines that would govern the way nurses expanded their roles. The focus on tasks was replaced by a view of nursing as a holistic caring activity, and the twin concepts of autonomy and accountability were introduced as the key to role expansion. These concepts have been discussed in depth by Walsh (2000), who points out that, as autonomous is synonymous with independence, it is a relative concept in the NHS. Nobody is fully autonomous, but we can enjoy higher levels of autonomy than we have in the past. Removing nursing tasks from medical delegation is clearly increasing the level of autonomy enjoyed by nurses. Accountability simply means being able to give an account of your actions. Nurses were therefore allowed to expand their role, provided that they could justify and explain their actions and also provided that they remained within the *Code of Professional Conduct*. They were also reminded that existing care should not suffer as a result of role expansion. In other words, if a nurse stopped carrying out a certain activity in order to create the time to expand their role, that activity had to be taken on by another appropriately qualified nurse.

The UKCC rightly stressed the need for education and training to underpin role expansion, and stated that individual nurses would be held responsible for ensuring that they were properly prepared for any new development they undertook.

The foundation stone of the *Code of Professional Conduct* is the primacy of the patient. Consequently, nurses needed to demonstrate that the rationale for role expansion was that it was in the patient's best interests. The primacy of the patient also means that nurses have to be fully competent to expand their role, especially as this involves increasing degrees of autonomy. Competency involves knowing the theory behind an action as well as being able to carry out the action effectively. It also involves knowing when to carry out an action that requires assessment and decision-making skills. By definition this takes nurses beyond the comfort zone of traditional pre-registration nursing education, otherwise it would not be role expansion. The UKCC, without seeming to realize it at the time, made it inevitable that nurses would have to acquire assessment and diagnostic skills that traditionally had been the preserve of medicine, if they were to expand their practice in accordance with the UKCC guidelines. The principles of accountability and autonomy enshrined within the *Scope of Professional Practice* document, when combined with other changes taking place within the NHS in the 1990s, made nurse practitioner development inevitable.

General managers and doctors may not be familiar with the contents of the *Scope of Professional Practice* or the *Code of Professional Conduct* documents. It is essential therefore that nurses who are involved in setting up nurse practitioner schemes make sure the implications of these two documents are fully explored and acted upon. They may be summarized by stating that a new advanced nursing role should only be introduced if:

- It is being done primarily for the benefit of patients
- Other aspects of patient care do not suffer as a result of role expansion
- The nurse is provided with education that is fit for purpose for the new role
- The role is seen holistically as an integrated development of nursing care rather than one or more isolated tasks that anybody could be trained to carry out
- The nurse is allowed the level of autonomy that is consistent with full accountability.

This last point is especially important. It is not possible to be fully accountable for your actions if you are not allowed a large amount of freedom of action. Put simply, there is no point in knowing what to do if you are not allowed to do it!

The nurse practitioner role today

It is essential to have a clear view of what the nurse practitioner role involves, for only in this way is it possible to look at the needs of the service and determine whether a nurse practitioner is the solution to the problem. As the UKCC refuse to recognize the nurse practitioner concept, we have to look to our North American colleagues for assistance.

An early and simple definition is that of Bliss and Cohen (1997), who stated that a nurse practitioner can assess the health care needs of the patient, carry out the whole range of health care interventions needed to meet those needs (including counselling), and collaborate with other health care agencies. This inclusive definition is underpinned by a strong, holistic nursing philosophy incorporating the psycho-social needs of the patient. It is also a very primary care-based definition. However, such an approach to care is being taken by many nurses working in A&E and minor injuries units, community hospitals and outpatients departments. Inpatient care is becoming more nurse-led in many areas, however, with medical consultants increasingly adopting the literal meaning of the title 'consultant' as nurses draw upon their expertise for advice in patient care. Bliss and Cohen therefore offer a simple definition that has a substantial amount of validity for the hospital role.

A more current and detailed definition comes from the American Nursing Association (ANA, 1996), and has arisen after considerable debate about the clinical nurse specialist and nurse practitioner roles. The term 'advanced practice nurse' is used to cover four different roles within the North American hospital system, of which the nurse practitioner is one. The others are the clinical nurse specialist, nurse-midwife and nurse-anaesthetist. Hickey (2000) points out that the advanced practice nurse carries out many of the activities involved in basic nursing practice, but the ANA definition shows where he or she has advanced their role beyond the basic registered nurse (RN). According to the ANA, the distinguishing features of advanced practice nurses when compared to RNs are that they:

- Manage patients with a greater depth and breadth of knowledge, skills and competencies
- Possess greater skills in managing organizations, systems of care and care environments
- Practise with greater autonomy
- Exercise a higher degree of independent judgement
- Use well-developed communication skills with multidisciplinary teams across complex health care environments.

In considering the four roles that are covered by this general advanced practice nurse definition, it should be noted that the midwife has already a well-established unique role in the National Health Service and nurse-anaesthetists do not really exist in the sense that they do in the USA. In fact, a simple way of getting strangers to the nurse practitioner role to understand it better is to liken it to that of the UK midwife, only in a nursing context.

Hospital-based nurse practitioners are covered by this broad advanced practice nurse definition, but in addition are seen as expert clinicians involved in the direct management of patient care (Hickey, 2000). They are able to carry out comprehensive assessments (including medical history taking and utilizing physical examination skills), make a diagnosis and prescribe both pharmacological and non-pharmacological therapeutic interventions, and are responsible for evaluating the effectiveness of their care. Their case load includes patients with both chronic and acute illnesses, and great emphasis is placed upon health promotion, health education and disease prevention. Emphasis is also placed upon working with families and whole communities as well as individual patients in order to achieve these goals.

This North American view stresses the importance of high levels of autonomy and has major implications for education, which will be discussed in Chapter 9. In the UK there is concern about the use of the word 'diagnosis', which is seen as an activity that only doctors can carry out. Consequently some nurses oppose the nurse practitioner concept on the grounds that is abandoning the nursing philosophy and selling out to medicine, whilst some doctors consider this is tantamount to nurses invading medical territory and usurping a fundamental medical function. However, a car mechanic 'diagnoses' what is wrong with a car, a central heating engineer 'diagnoses' what is wrong with a boiler, and a television football pundit 'diagnoses' why a favourite club just cannot seem to win matches. The term therefore has a much wider meaning and is about working out what a problem is and giving it a label. That label is the diagnosis. Nurses need not therefore fear that nurse practitioners are abandoning nursing simply because they use a term such as diagnosis, since all they are doing is working out what is wrong with the patient and giving it a label.

The medical profession has perhaps more of a case to argue when it accuses nurse practitioners of treading on medical territory by using the word diagnosis. It is true that it takes a great deal of expertise to arrive at many medical diagnoses, but it is also true that it does not need the brains of Einstein to diagnose a laceration of the thumb or a sprained ankle. As long as nurse practitioners remain within the basic principles of the *Scope of Professional Practice* and accept full accountability for their actions, they will restrain their diagnostic activity to those areas where they are competent by virtue of their educational preparation for the role and their experience.

Diagnostics is not an all-or-nothing concept where only medical practitioners can diagnose anything at all and no other person is capable of any diagnostic function. In many cases the diagnostic expert is the patient. Doctors have been known to get diagnoses wrong on occasion! The growth of algorithms, increasingly sophisticated diagnostic equipment and computer-assisted diagnostic techniques have all served to remove the mystique surrounding diagnosis. It is time to rethink our approach to this word diagnosis and to adopt a more flexible approach. No nurse practitioner would attempt a complex diagnosis such as multiple sclerosis. However, nurse practitioners are capable of diagnosing many conditions and acting accordingly, whilst they are also capable of using the same skills to narrow down the range of possible diagnoses and ensure that a patient receives appropriate medical attention when it is needed. Accident and emergency nurses have been undertaking this latter function, here known as triage, for many years, whilst the growth of NHS Direct is based upon the same principle. Paramedics encountering

seriously injured or ill patients many miles from hospital have to diagnose what is going on in order to respond appropriately. Perhaps it is better to say that medicine makes the definitive diagnosis, especially where the pathology is complex, but that there are many situations where a 'working diagnosis' of what is probably wrong has to be made without a medical presence. There are also other cases where an appropriately trained nurse practitioner or paramedic could equally well make the diagnosis. Diagnosis can no longer be claimed to be the exclusive prerogative of medicine.

The final definition of the nurse practitioner role that needs to be introduced is the only one proposed by a major national UK nursing body, the RCN. In 1996 the RCN Council issued a position statement that the role of nurse practitioners is to:

- See patients with undifferentiated and undiagnosed problems as the first point of contact
- Make a health assessment using extra skills not normally taught in nursing education to date
- Make professionally autonomous decisions for which they have sole responsibility
- Develop a plan of nursing care to promote health
- Provide counselling and health education for patients
- Screen patients for early signs of illness and risk factors
- Have the authority to refer patients to other health professionals or admit/discharge if appropriate.

The RCN also added that the minimum educational standard for the role was Honours degree level.

This role description is the basis for the RCNI course and therefore relates education to preparation for the role. The RCN definition is close to the widely accepted North American view, stressing that nurse practitioners are the first point of contact and that they will therefore have to use extra skills (e.g. physical assessment and history taking) in their assessment before arriving at a judgement concerning patients' problems. The word diagnosis is tactfully avoided in this definition, but the emphasis on health promotion, health education, counselling skills and a plan of nursing care all ensure that nurses are reminded that however much they are expanding their role, they are still practising as nurses.

The RCN role description fits the hospital role well. We have taught nurse practitioners working in A&E, minor injuries, surgical pre-assessment, outpatients, emergency admissions units and inpatient areas, including critical care. Patients attending A&E obviously have undifferentiated and undiagnosed problems, as do patients in acute medical or surgical admission units. Patients who are being managed by nurse practitioners on an outpatient basis also fit these criteria. A great deal can have happened to a patient since seeing the consultant 6 months ago, so when they present to the nurse practitioner, he or she needs to be sure that there are no other serious new problems developing whilst helping the patient to cope with known problems. A similar observation applies to nurse practitioners working in a surgical pre-admission role, whose main concern is working up patients for list surgery and ensuring a smooth post-operative discharge. Nurse practitioners working within a specialist field whose role includes inpatients may also find themselves called to the ward by the nursing staff to assess a patient who has developed a new problem. Clinical specialities such as orthopaedics, urology, gynaecology, ENT, vascular surgery, colorectal surgery and fertility/assisted conception are all represented on our nurse practitioner programme at present, which demonstrates the wide range of specialist areas where a nurse practitioner role can be developed.

In order to help nurse practitioners to decide what the problems may be (make a diagnosis), they have to have the freedom to order relevant investigations such as radiographs or lab work. Hospital traditions that only doctors can order investigations have to be set aside and replaced by agreed ways of working which place the patients' best interests first. It is not in the patients' best interests to have to wait hours for a doctor to sign a piece of paper authorizing a simple lab test or radiograph. Once nurse practitioners have completed their assessment (diagnosis) they must be able to act according to how they see fit, which means that there must be greater degrees of autonomy built into the role. Nurse practitioners have to have the authority necessary to do the job, and negoti-

ations must take place in advance with the other 'teams and tribes' both in the hospital and outside to ensure that this is so. The final point in the RCN definition about referrals is crucial to the functioning of a hospital nurse practitioner.

A new skill that nurse practitioners will have to learn is the management of uncertainty. This is a particular skill that doctors learn from early on in their education but which has been absent from nursing education. In making a diagnosis, the doctor, and hence nurse practitioner, is usually dealing in probabilities rather than certainties. It is dangerous to foreclose too early in the diagnostic process and come to a single definitive decision about what is wrong with the patient. Other avenues have to be explored, double checks carried out, second opinions sought and further investigations considered, and sometimes the best thing to do is nothing at all as time alone may reveal what is really happening.

Evidence and the benefits of the nurse practitioner role

In this modern era of evidence-based practice it is right to ask 'What does the evidence about the nurse practitioner role tell us?'. The evidence is very positive, and most of the following chapters contain examples of research into various nurse practitioner developments. The evidence in support of the nurse practitioner is so strong that perhaps today we are guilty of asking the wrong question. Rather than asking 'Is the nurse practitioner role effective?', perhaps we should be asking 'Why is the nurse practitioner role so effective?'. Extensive North American research exists supporting the nurse practitioner role, and there is a steadily growing UK body of evidence that is also very positive.

The Coopers and Lybrand Report (1996) is a good introduction to this body of research evidence. The findings of this study are typical of many smaller scale pieces of research, and act as a good introductory summary to the evidence base underpinning the nurse practitioner role. The Coopers and Lybrand study looked at 10 different nurse practitioner roles, four of which were based in hospital outpatients departments and one in a community hospital, and one that provided a hospital outreach service to drug addicts and prostitutes. The other nurse practitioner roles were generalist nurse practitioners in community settings.

The study showed considerable improvements in access to services and the speed with which patients were seen. Patients also commented very favourably about the ease with which they could understand information and advice given, especially when compared with conventional medical advice. Other health staff found their workloads reduced and that they had more time as a result of newly established nurse practitioner services. Costing the projects proved very difficult in practice, but the report concluded that there was firm evidence of equal or better levels of output and quality at reduced costs at six of the sites, while there was insufficient evidence available at the remaining four sites to make any statement about costs. The report mentions many benefits that could not be costed, such as better interdisciplinary teamwork, a more holistic approach to care, crossing primary/secondary health care boundaries, and more rapid access to services. Nurse practitioner-led services were seen as innovative and, given the need to reform and renew the NHS, this observation is particularly important.

One final key benefit of nurse practitioner services was that they greatly improved job satisfaction for the nurses involved. The prime reason for introducing the nurse practitioner role has to be the primacy of the patient and improving standards of care. However, we cannot ignore the fact that one of the major problems facing the NHS today is the retention of skilled and experienced nursing staff, and any initiative that enhances the job satisfaction of such staff therefore has to be seen as a positive move. Improving job satisfaction and hence retention rates for experienced nursing staff is therefore a likely major bonus of developing a nurse practitioner service.

The report concluded that nurse practitioners offer an intrinsically different service to medicine and that they are not 'doctors on the cheap'. Many benefits were identified, both for the patient and for other health care staff. However, there were problems stemming from lack of understanding of the nurse practitioner role by other professionals, confusion over boundaries, insufficient support staff, and lack

of provision for absences. The report also noted a tendency for patients to be more impressed by the doctor's traditional authority than by the nurse practitioner. Coopers and Lybrand (1996) speculated that this might translate into better compliance with 'doctor's orders' rather than the nurse practitioner's health education advice. This is an important issue, which will be returned to later, and hinges on whether patients are seen as passive recipients or active partners in care.

The following key factors were seen by Coopers and Lybrand (1996) as helping to establish and maintain nurse practitioner-led services:

- Establishing good communications with other staff and a support network for nurse practitioners
- Establishing the need for the nurse practitioner service and the level of provision required with other health staff
- Identifying the educational and clinical supervision requirements of nurse practitioners in order that they may deliver the level of service decided upon
- Recognizing that the role is dynamic and allowing for growth and change in setting up the service
- Establishing clinical guidelines and protocols so that all concerned are aware of how nurse practitioners are working, and the nurse practitioners know they are following best practice with the full support of the Trust
- Ensuring that the project is properly planned and evaluated, with the nurse practitioner a key member of the management group
- Recognizing the fact that there will be barriers to such a new way of working, and that these barriers have to be identified and time and resources invested by the Trust in overcoming them.

A moment's reflection on the complex structures and systems of working that characterize a modern hospital will show that the above list is extremely relevant and represents good-quality evidence upon which to base development of nurse practitioner services. There has to be a clear rationale and identified service need that has been thought through before a nurse practitioner service is established. Important factors such as the level of service provision, cost and clinical effectiveness can then be considered with key interrelated topics such as quality, clinical governance and evaluation of the role. These can then be teased out and integrated into the project, together with medico-legal and professional role boundary issues. These issues are complex but need to be worked through before nurse practitioner services are established, and they will be explored in more detail in the next chapter.

Conclusion

This chapter has introduced many of the key issues involved in implementing the nurse practitioner role within the hospital setting, including the basic tenet that the nurse practitioner role is primarily about improving patient care rather than cutting costs or implementing government directives on junior doctors' hours. Nurse practitioners must have a fit for purpose education to prepare them for the role, and success depends upon good interdisciplinary teamworking with all professionals. We have explored the basic role definition and its focus on seeing patients with undifferentiated and undiagnosed health problems and deriving a plan of care from that initial assessment, which is carried out with higher levels of autonomy and accountability than has been the case traditionally in nursing. Not only have we a lot to learn from the growth of the role in North America, but we could also learn lessons a lot nearer home from the way midwifery colleagues have developed their profession. The evidence base for the nurse practitioner role is very strong in the USA and is growing stronger all the time in the UK. The rest of this book is dedicated to a fuller exploration of many of these issues, and should leave the reader ready and able to seize the tremendous opportunities offered by the nurse

practitioner role in developing our NHS for a new century. It is axiomatic, however, that the old borderlines have to be redrawn as the nurse practitioner role develops and emerges on the existing boundaries between medicine and nursing.

References

ANA (1996). *Scope and Standards of Advanced Practice Registered Nursing.* American Nursing Association.

Bacon, F. (1640). *De Dignitate et Augmentis Scientarium*, **I, vi,** 31 *Antitheta*, 6 (trans. Gilbert Watts).

Bliss, A. and Cohen, E. (1997). The New Health Professionals Nurse Practitioner and Physicians Assistant. Aspen Publications, Colorado.

Coopers and Lybrand (1996). *Nurse Practitioner Evaluation Summary.* Coopers and Lybrand Health Practice.

DHSS (1977). *The Extended Role of the Nurse.* Department of Health and Social Security.

Hickey, J. (2000). Advanced practice nursing at the dawn of the 21st century: practice education and research. In: *Advanced Practice Nursing*, 2nd edn (J. Hickey, R. Oumiette and S. Venegoni, eds), Lippincott.

Mitchell, J. (1994). *Borderline.* Turbulent Indigo. Reprise Records.

Proehl, J. (2000). Respice, prospice, looking forward and looking back. Plenary Paper. *Emergency Nursing 2000 and Beyond. International Conference in Emergency Care.* Royal College of Nursing Edinburgh.

Running, A., Calder, J., Mustain, B. and Foreschier, C. (2000). A survey of nurse practitioners across the United States. *Nurse Practitioner*, **25,** 6, 15–16, 110–116.

UKCC (1992). *Scope of Professional Practice.* UKCC.

Walsh, M. (2000). *Nursing Frontiers; Accountability and the Boundaries of Care.* Butterworth-Heinemann, Oxford.

2

THE NURSE PRACTITIONER ROLE IN HOSPITAL: PROFESSIONAL AND ORGANIZATIONAL ISSUES

Mike Walsh

History is always more comfortable
Than the implications of the present.
Alan Bold (1985)

Introduction

Today is the present, and the today on which I am writing this chapter is a few weeks after the publication of the Government's National Health Service (NHS) Plan (DoH, 2000). The plan has immense implications for the NHS in England that will be uncomfortable for many. The other three countries in the United Kingdom cannot ignore the plan, and its implications will therefore extend across the UK as a whole. Change is uncomfortable, and there may therefore be a strong temptation in some quarters to find reasons for not changing anything and continuing to live in history. All staff working in the NHS have a collective responsibility to recognize that we have to radically change the NHS if it is to survive, however uncomfortable that may be. The resources are now promised, together with a government that appears to have the political will to make those changes. The nature of the changes being proposed have immense implications for nursing and patient care, and make the further development of the nurse practitioner role in hospitals even more likely if Labour's promises are to be delivered.

By the time you study this page, it is likely that there will have been a general election. Public opinion polls in the summer of 2000 indicate that it is likely that the existing Labour government will win that election and will therefore be implementing the NHS 2000 Plan, or at least something very similar. The implications of this plan for nurse practitioner development therefore need to be explored if we are to see the big picture or context within which each of us will practise. It is of course possible that the general election might have produced a major upset and returned a Tory government. That does not render this introduction invalid, however, as the Tory party has itself recognized the need for a major overhaul of the NHS, which must involve expanding nursing roles.

The NHS Plan

The announcement of this major government initiative was actually made by the Prime Minister in the House of Commons, rather than the Secretary of State for Health, which demonstrates the importance of the plan to the Labour government. It was a far-reaching and comprehensive document, which repeatedly stressed the need to improve access to and speed up the delivery of health care. We have already seen in the preceding chapter that research into the nurse practitioner role has consistently shown that it achieves both these targets, whether in the primary health care or the hospital environment. An example of this approach is the statement in the NHS Plan that by 2004 no patient should wait in accident and emergency departments for more than 4 hours from arrival to admission, transfer or discharge. Fast-track nurse practitioner-led services will make a major contribution to meeting this goal.

The government has also pledged 500 NHS Walk-In Centres for rapid access to health care, whilst NHS Direct is another attempt to make health care more accessible. Nurses are heavily involved in both these schemes, and the assessment and clinical decision-making skills of the nurse practitioner are well to the fore in making either scheme work. The alternative is increasing dependence upon computer software and protocols that reduce nurses to the level of button pressers. Both these initiatives have significant implications for the hospital sector, particularly accident and emergency and admissions units to which some patients will be referred. Nurse practitioners may therefore be referring patients from a primary care setting to fellow nurse practitioners in hospital.

The NHS Plan promises 7000 extra beds by 2004, 2100 of which will be in acute wards and 4900 in intermediate care. When the provision of extra beds is linked to the reduction in junior doctors' hours, it is clear that staffing those beds is going to be a major headache. The promise of 20 000 new nurses is encouraging but is unlikely to make any impact upon staffing these extra beds in the short to medium term. It takes several years to recruit and educate nurses, assuming that the recruits can be found in the first place. It takes even longer for those registered nurses to become proficient practitioners, as they need hard-won experience and further education to develop beyond basic competence. It takes even longer to recruit and train doctors. The NHS Plan promises 7500 extra hospital consultants, but the first of those extra consultants will be unlikely to be taking up their posts until well into the second decade of this new century.

If the government is to open up over 2000 acute hospital beds by 2004 it needs an immediate solution to a major staffing problem, which will not be found in the plan's promise of new medical and nursing recruits. We need to find new ways of working in hospitals that make better use of the staff who are already there, and which improves retention rates as well as bringing ex-nurses back into practice. The nurse practitioner concept can make a major contribution to the challenge of caring for more patients in more beds with basically the same staffing levels. The Coopers and Lybrand (1996) report stresses that nurse practitioner roles greatly improve nurses' job satisfaction, and this should have a beneficial effect upon retention. However, a shift in attitudes is required towards traditional medical and nursing boundaries if this possibility is to be realized. This point is well made by Hunter (2000), who points out that the NHS is not homogeneous, as there are '... multiple tribes each with its own values and culture'. He goes on to urge the need for recognition of these differences, and then support and assistance for the champions of change within each NHS tribe. Otherwise, he concludes, '...sustainable long term change will elude us all'.

The issue of tribalism within the NHS has already been introduced in Chapter 1, and there is a danger that a centralized plan such as that proposed may overlook the fractured and fragmented nature of the NHS that actually exists on the ground. All the good intentions may therefore come to nothing. To move forwards, nursing must embrace the nurse practitioner concept and at the same time work collaboratively with the other professional 'tribes' of the NHS to overcome the inevitable boundary problems that will occur. Nursing must first however put its own house in order and put an end to the internal squabbling exemplified by health visitors' reported complaints over the government's decision to drop the title Health Visitor from nursing's new Regulatory Body (Nursing Standard, 2000). Ultimately, we are all nurses.

The provision of over 4000 extra intermediate care beds presents another major staffing challenge, which nurse practitioners are well suited to meet. It is likely that many of the patients in these beds will be elderly and recovering from an episode of acute illness superimposed on long-term chronic health problems. There is a rapidly growing body of North American evidence to suggest that the nurse practitioner offers a high-quality, cost-effective key to the management of patients in the post-acute care period (Rapp, 2000).

Curtin and Lubkin (1998) describe acute illness as being like unexpected visitors who leave one's house after a short-term visit. Their arrival is sudden and they may cause major upset to the equilibrium of the household, but eventually they leave. Chronic illness, however, lingers and is a continual part of the person's life and environment. Intermediate care beds offer a transition from the acute illness to the chronic resting state, and have the obvious advantage of freeing up acute hospital beds for those most in need of immediate care. However, the patient at this stage still has significant medical problems in need of on-going assessment and management in addition to their nursing care needs; hence the relevance of the nurse practitioner care. Nurse practitioners must of course be able to refer a patient back to a hospital doctor and an acute bed rapidly should their condition deteriorate. Rapp (2000) provides a lucid account of how the nurse practitioner may work in this intermediate care environment, spanning the gap between acute ward and community care. She cites extensive North American evidence showing that the main reason doctors give for having to readmit patients to acute beds is that nurses lack appropriate assessment skills to monitor the medical progress of the patient. This is compounded by an inability to communicate information effectively concerning an acute change in condition. Rapp (2000) considers that nurse practitioners provide the bridge that will carry the patient over this post-acute area, as they can bring together the findings from an holistic nursing assessment with the symptom-focused physical examination and medical history. If during intermediate care the patient's condition changes significantly for the worse, the nurse practitioner can then perform a symptom-based assessment, formulate a differential diagnosis and present the patient to a senior hospital doctor quickly, concisely and in language that the doctor understands. The result is intermediate care that does not absorb scarce medical resources but is safe for the patient as, should any problems develop, they can either be managed by the nurse practitioner or rapidly referred for medical management in an acute ward.

The model of working outlined above and shown diagrammatically in Figure 2.1 can be applied to a range of hospital settings in addition to intermediate care, and shows how the nurse practitioner brings together the practice of nursing and medicine to produce something that is a powerful hybrid of both. Figure 2.1 shows the direct 'Route One' approach of medicine, homing in on the chief complaint and working through to a diagnosis via history taking and a physical exam, integrated with the holistic nursing model, which is concerned with the human response to health and illness. A key treatment option in this scenario is medical referral. This means that doctors in other specialities need to be prepared to accept referrals direct from nurse practitioners rather than going through the third party of a doctor within a nurse practitioner's speciality. It is only fair, however, to expect nurse practitioners to demonstrate their competence in differential diagnosis and decision making before such a system is established. This underlines the importance of degree-level education for the nurse practitioner role. The model shown in Figure 2.1

could equally well work in a surgical pre-admission unit, an emergency medical admission unit or an inpatient speciality area such as ENT or urology.

The NHS Plan also envisages that nurses will have more powers to prescribe, refer, admit and discharge patients. These are all aspects of the nurse practitioner role definition explored in Chapter 1 and which fit the model outlined above. If the government is serious about this kind of expansion in nursing roles, it has to be serious about the nurse practitioner.

Changing the hospital system

There is a great deal of frustration amongst nurse practitioners at the intransigent attitude displayed by national nursing authorities toward their development, and also at the major struggle involved in changing the culture of hospitals which restricts nursing development. However, change is possible, and the next section of this chapter will explore key factors involved in changing the system.

A very important lesson can be learnt from the success achieved by North American nurses in campaigning to change legislation to allow direct Medicare reimbursement for Advanced Practice Nurses (APNs). The operational details of the Medicare system are obviously not relevant to the UK; however, an analysis of how after years of frustration APNs achieved this major breakthrough, which improves access to health care for many in the USA, is very illuminating. Wong (1999) states that the success was due to nurses uniting and overcoming their tendency to fragment. Working together, they were able to influence legislation that led directly to improvements in patient care. Wong (1999) also provides an insightful analysis of the politics involved in making this major change, which holds valid lessons for nurses in the UK.

The work of Kingdon (1995) is used as an analytical framework by Wong (1999). Kingdon argues that policy formation in a democratic government involves interaction between participants and the problem together with the politics and policy that relate to that problem. When a policy is turned into legislation, these factors all come together and an opportunity exists to influence the formu-

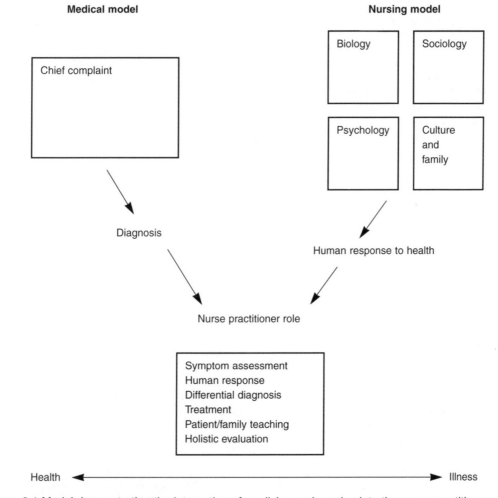

Medical model

Chief complaint

Diagnosis

Nursing model

Biology

Sociology

Psychology

Culture and family

Human response to health

Nurse practitioner role

Symptom assessment
Human response
Differential diagnosis
Treatment
Patient/family teaching
Holistic evaluation

Health ←—————————————————————————→ Illness

Figure 2.1 Model demonstrating the integration of medicine and nursing into the nurse practitioner role in hospital care (adapted from Rapp, 2000).

lation of that policy. The complex problem facing the USA government was the need to combine reducing the budget deficit with providing cost-effective health care, and the combination of these twin problems created an opportunity that APNs were able to exploit. The Labour government in the UK (and indeed any future Tory government) faces a similar problem of controlling public expenditure but also improving the NHS. The parallels are therefore striking.

Wong (1999) states that nurses should first identify the key participants. Bill Clinton, President of the USA, was seen as far more important than Federal officials in her analysis.

This approach indicates that nurses seeking to pursue the policy of expanding nursing roles should target the Prime Minister and Health Secretary for England, together with key politicians in devolved government elsewhere in the UK.

Politics is about the exercise of power. Wong (1999) states this includes public opinion, government, organized political parties and elections. Evaluation of the nurse practitioner role consistently shows that it is very favourably viewed by the general public once they understand what it involves (Coopers and Lybrand, 1996). This favourable public opinion should not however be taken for granted, as the recent series of scandals involving doctors has badly damaged their image in the eyes of the general public and the slipped halo effect may tend to raise doubts about all health staff. One or two well-publicized nurse practitioner errors that led to serious patient harm could have a disastrous effect upon public opinion, which is notoriously fickle.

The Labour government elected in 1997 has taken nursing far more seriously than any of its predecessors. A further favourable sign was the way the Tory leader William Hague effectively invited himself to address the annual RCN Congress in Bournemouth in 2000, indicating that his party perhaps now considers nursing to be more important than it did when in government. The NHS is always a major issue in UK general elections, and with one in the offing in the next 18 months it can be seen that the key factors involved in the political process are all in place and running in the nurse practitioners' favour at present.

Nursing must exploit this opportunity to show that nurse practitioners can make a major contribution to solving the problem of saving the NHS, and doing so in a cost-effective way. We need organizations such as the Royal College of Nursing (RCN) to use the evidence showing the benefits of the nurse practitioner, to lobby with a united voice. The same exercise can also take place locally if nurses follow the strategy of identifying the key personnel and showing how the policy of developing nurse practitioner services can solve local problems. A key issue nationally is whether the government, once persuaded of the efficacy of the nurse practitioner, is prepared to bring pressure to bear upon the UKCC or its successor to promote nurse practitioner recognition.

A major step in successful lobbying is to market the nurse practitioner role and to do so with hard evidence. Wong (1999) cites evidence from the US Office of Technology Assessment showing that up to 80 per cent of primary health care can be delivered by nurse practitioners to the same or better quality standards and at lower costs as being crucial in winning the argument. However, it was the presentation of this kind of evidence by a united nursing profession at the right time, when there was a confluence of problem, policy and politics, that led to a positive outcome.

There is a further striking parallel with the situation in the USA. Wong (1999) observes that when a provision appears as a small part of a larger bill, it has far more chance of success. Government support for the nurse practitioner role can be seen as a small part of the much bigger NHS rebuilding plan. The same logic applies, and should therefore be exploited to promote the nurse practitioner role as a small but essential part of solving the problem of resuscitating the NHS. Nursing unity is however essential to achieving progress, and Wong issues a crucial warning about the dangers of intra-professional rivalry when she observes (Wong, 1999, p. 172):

What is the value of disputing whether clinical nurse specialists should have the same privileges as nurse practitioners? Are we trying to influence health policy to be able to provide more access to holistic, high-quality care or are we simply trying to advance our own ambitions?

Power and the nurse practitioner

The above analysis revolves around power and its exercise in the political arena. We should therefore turn our attention to how the nurse practitioner should address the inevitable issues of power in the hospital setting.

A straightforward view of power is that it is something that is derived either from the position a person holds in the hospital, or that it is personal and derived from the individual in some way (La Monica, 1990). The former arises when superior authority delegates power to a person (e.g. appoints someone as a manager of a unit) by right of office (it is in the job description!), or it arises out of the person's expertise and knowledge. Position power therefore flows downwards. Personal power flows upwards, and comes from the willingness of people to be led by another person. This in turn depends upon good interpersonal communication skills, possessing valued characteristics such as being easy to get on with and expertise. La Monica suggests that a nursing leader should be able to draw upon both sources of power. If nurse practitioners are to be seen as leaders of nursing, this suggests that they must be visibly delegated a measure of authority from higher management, and that this should be written in their job description. This might include the authority to order radiographs or refer patients to medical colleagues. However, nurse practitioners will also obtain the power necessary to enable them to carry out their role through good interpersonal and communication skills and, above all, demonstrable clinical expertise. These characteristics will earn the respect of both medical and nursing colleagues, the latter being particularly important if nurse practitioners are to have the co-operation and support of their registered nurse colleagues. The combination of a good educational preparation and clinical experience are therefore essential prerequisites for nurse practitioner role development.

A more subtle analysis of power sees it as dispersed throughout the fabric of any society. It is often disguised, operating through a series of relationships, practices and systems that are frequently covert. There may also be localized centres of power that are not so covert. One of the key implications of this analysis is that although it is possible to change the macro-structure of a society, this will have little effect upon the power structures because they are ingrained in the woodwork and are concerned with the way people relate to each other (Peterson and Bunton, 1997). This analysis of power is derived from the work of Foucault (Peterson and Bunton, 1997), and is immediately recognizable in any hospital. Hospital management may attempt to restructure a unit (the 'macrostructure' of Peterson and Bunton), but if nurse practitioners are really to develop the potential of their role, inter-personal relationships with other key professionals, not just doctors, hold the key.

Reveley (1999) has shown the importance of understanding how power is traditionally distributed between staff, and how this affects interpersonal relationships and influences differing perspectives on developing the nurse practitioner role. Her research utilized the negotiated order perspective first proposed by Strauss *et al.* (1963) and applied to the relationship between medicine and nursing by writers such as Svensson (1996). This work is concerned with how social orders are negotiated, maintained and adapted to fit the changing circumstances within which people live. Such negotiations take place in a patterned and systematic fashion, and are essentially a mix of the organization's rules and informal understandings regulating the relationships between different groups of people on a day-to-day basis. There are two key insights that the negotiated order perspective has for nurse practitioners. First, the balance of power between different groups of staff may shift and change in response to changing circumstances. It is therefore continually subject to renegotiation, and the *status quo* can be altered. The second point to remember is that different groups of staff will interpret the same situation differently, and as a result construct their own meanings from events. Doctors will tend to interpret the nurse practitioner concept differently from nurses, for example; therefore both parties have to clarify and understand each other's perceptions of the concept if agreement is to be reached.

The key power relationship for the nurse practitioner is that between medicine and nursing, as medicine has to relinquish a degree of its power if the nurse practitioner is to develop. Reveley (1999) applied this theoretical insight to her study of nurse practitioner role introduction, and found convincing evidence of nurse practitioners and doctors actually renegotiating their roles as nurse practitioners became involved in diagnosis and treatment decisions. The balance of power shifted away from the doctors as nurse practitioners demonstrated their learning and increased competence, with the result that the relationship became increasingly one of monitoring rather than direct supervision. Increasing levels of autonomy developed gradually, and had to be earned and negotiated over time. Nurse practitioner role development is therefore a continually evolving product of negotiation with the medical profession, based upon demonstrated competence. The hospital nurse practitioner role should therefore not be envisaged as something that starts with a 'big bang', but as one that evolves out of growing confidence and mutual respect on the part of medicine and nursing as the role develops, allowing a negotiated expansion in nursing autonomy. For those who are critical of this approach on the grounds that it places medicine in a dominant position, we can only say, welcome to reality! Medicine is the dominant paradigm in health care, and nurse practitioners have to work with medical colleagues towards a negotiated shift in the way things are done. In this way we can maintain the great benefits of medical practice, but add the extra benefits that nursing can bring to patient care. The result, of course, is the nurse practitioner.

A further key observation of Foucault (cited in Petersen and Bunton, 1997) is the famous dictum that knowledge is power; an increase in one brings about an increase in the other. This links to the analysis presented by La Monica (1990), who sees knowledge and expertise underpinning both positional and personal power. The graduate nurse practitioner who can talk knowledgeably the language of differential diagnosis and symptom analysis has a far greater chance of earning the respect of doctors and, ultimately, the authority that is associated with real power.

Nurse practitioners should not however be seeking power for the sake of it. A criticism often levelled at medicine is that it is a means of social control (Foucault, cited in Petersen and Bunton, 1997), whilst Davies (1996) was very critical of what she called male-dominated, old-style nineteenth century professions such as medicine, which are characterized by power-seeking behaviour. This male characteristic of seeking power in order to dominate others is contrasted by Davies with the more collaborative model advocated by feminists, who argue that power is for sharing. A telling comment was made by the former RCN President, Dame June Clark, when she observed that the power of nursing lies in giving power away (Hancock, 2000). The essence of Clark's observation is that nursing is immensely powerful because it can share power with other nurses, and above all with the patient and family, rather than hoarding power as the currency of expertise. Patient education and health promotion are key aspects of the nurse practitioner role, and they are all about sharing knowledge with patients in order to empower them.

If knowledge leads to power, the legitimate exercise of that power constitutes authority. However, power that is not recognized as legitimate is coercion (Wilkinson and Miers, 1999), and has no part in the ethical practice of nursing. Authority is essential for the practice of nurse practitioners and therefore their power has to be recognized as legitimate. In setting up a nurse practitioner role,

exploration of all the issues with key staff in advance is essential to legitimize the power that the nurse practitioner will possess. Good educational preparation and clinical experience will also legitimize the role.

Without authority nurses cannot be held truly accountable for their actions, and without the necessary authority to fulfil the role the nurse practitioner will quickly become frustrated. In establishing a new nurse practitioner role it is therefore essential at the beginning to map out the authority the nurse practitioner will need to carry out that role. The linkage between power and authority should not be forgotten, together with the observation that power can only be demonstrated through behaviour (La Monica, 1990). A refusal to grant appropriate authority to the nurse practitioner is tantamount to a refusal to share power. Conversely, nurse practitioners should remember that the power and hence authority that they are granted will only be maintained by their behaviour in their role. The socialization of women into self-effacing, loyal subordinates makes it difficult for many female nurse practitioners to get used to the exercise of power. However, the notice in a local village post office window under threat of closure makes the point: 'Use it or lose it!' The need is for a quiet assertiveness rather than a strident approach reminiscent of Margaret Thatcher.

In summary, therefore, power stems both from the positions held by nurse practitioners within the hospital and from their own personal characteristics and ability to get others to follow their lead. Knowledge and expertise are fundamental aspects of power, but there are also covert power systems in any organization that stem from interpersonal relationships. Authority is essential for nurse practitioners, and that authority is no more than the legitimate exercise of their power; however, if power is not used it will also be lost and with it the nurse practitioner's authority. Above all, nurses should use power more constructively than other predominantly male groups have in the past. Power has to be won to allow the nurse practitioner to function, but can then be shared with patients as part of the nurse practitioner's therapeutic role.

Power is a necessary part of change, and change has to occur if the nurse practitioner role is to be implemented. It is essential, however, that nurses play a major part in leading such change rather than reacting passively to the initiatives of others. The literature on change is very substantial, and has been reviewed in the light of nursing development by Walsh (2000). The following key points and their implications for nurse practitioner roles in hospitals may be distilled from this review.

Change should be bottom up, utilizing the principles of the normative–educative approach

The need for the nurse practitioner role should arise from the everyday experiences of staff and patients, rather than be imposed from above by a manager who thinks it might be a good idea. If staff recognize the need for change and have the opportunity to explore what the nurse practitioner role involves, recognizing it as a potential solution to a problem, they are more likely to accept, own and support the implementation of the nurse practitioner role.

Opposition to change is more often due to staff's perceptions of the implications of change rather than the change itself

Medical staff may see nurse practitioners as interlopers intruding on medical territory or as cheap substitutes, either way undermining the medical profession. Alternatively, if nurse practitioners are seen as physicians' assistants they will be trained under a purely medical model, isolated from other nurses and given the tedious repetitive tasks that junior doctors do not wish to undertake. If patients see nurse practitioners as cheap substitutes for a doctor, the implications are that patients may lack confidence in them, undermining their practice. Fellow nurses who see nurse practitioners as elite 'supernurses' may be resentful and uncooperative. Negative implications such as these may all flow from a failure to assess properly the service level provision required in the first instance and then work through the meaning of the role with all staff involved. Misunderstandings about the role will therefore lead to resistance.

Lewin's Force Field analysis is a useful tool in implementing change

This simple tool (Lewin, 1951) involves drawing up a list of the factors that are either driving or opposing change. Once these have been identified, the *status quo* can be unfrozen and change occur by strengthening the drivers and weakening the opposition to change before finally re-freezing the situation in its changed form (i.e. after implementation of the nurse practitioner role).

Drivers for change include:

- Providing specific information about local practice rather than relying upon national statistics
- Identifying influential people such as senior doctors who are supportive of the nurse practitioner concept
- Forming a project team who meet regularly to see the nurse practitioner implementation through to successful evaluation
- Offering the introduction of the nurse practitioner as a reversible option
- Giving people the necessary education and training to work with the new nurse practitioner concept as well as the time to prepare for it
- Keeping all relevant staff fully informed about the nurse practitioner developments at all times.

Forces opposing change may be overcome if:

- Support from senior management for the nurse practitioner role is forthcoming
- The nurse practitioner change is seen to be internally driven rather than externally imposed
- There are obvious benefits to staff from introducing the nurse practitioner role
- There are guarantees that the introduction of the nurse practitioner does not undermine the job security or salary of others
- Introducing the nurse practitioner role is seen as an exciting and interesting opportunity
- There is good effective communication with all involved.

The ideas expressed above will serve as starters to get you thinking about what other drivers and opposers to change there may be in your area. Upsetting the balance of forces is essential to overcoming the *status quo* and introducing nurse practitioner-led changes.

Practice development such as the introduction of the nurse practitioner role is most likely to succeed when the three factors of evidence, context and facilitation are most favourable

Kitson *et al.* (1998) proposed a very attractive model that helps to explain successful practice development. Their work suggests that a strong evidence base for introducing the nurse practitioner role is an essential but not a sufficient condition. The context within which the nurse practitioner role is being introduced and how the change is facilitated are equally important, and the interaction of these two factors with the strength of the evidence base play a major role in determining outcome. A favourable context is one in which staff feel involved and valued, there is good communication, role clarity already exists, quality assurance work and feedback to staff about performance takes place, there are good inter-personal relationships and there is effective leadership. A facilitator who can think laterally, cross professional boundaries, be open-minded, confident, non-judgemental and supportive, and whose role is understood by all concerned, will also aid implementation of the nurse practitioner role. It is unreasonable to leave the nurse practitioner to 'get on with it' without the support of a facilitator, who could be a member of the local university staff, a practice development officer or a member of staff on secondment with the brief of helping to implement the nurse practitioner role. Trusts planning to introduce nurse practitioners should therefore search the evidence base carefully, optimize the context within which they will work, and use a facilitator to help implement the role. Good facilitation in a favourable context will greatly aid the renegoti-ation of power and relationships that has to take place between nursing and medicine for nurse practitioner role implementation.

Change always has to be seen within the strategic framework of the NHS

We have already seen how the juxtaposition of policy, politics and problems at governmental level can create opportunities for major changes (p. 14). Pettigrew *et al.* (1992) carried out significant research into change at strategic level in the NHS, and identified eight factors that promote change. They stress, however, that there is not a simple linear cause and effect relationship between each single factor and the probability of change; rather it is the interplay between the factors overall that influences the likelihood of change occurring. The eight factors are as follows.

1. *Environmental pressure.* Factors such as medical shortages, an ageing population, and government initiatives such as the NHS Plan (and the need for the Tory party to come up with a convincing alternative) ensure strong environmental pressure favouring the nurse practitioner concept.
2. *A supportive organizational culture.* Culture is again seen as crucial. Perhaps it is best to start introducing the role in those areas of your hospital which have a more change-friendly culture. This links back to the earlier discussion about context.
3. *Changing the agenda and its locale.* It is necessary to be clear what the real agenda is and from where the drive for change is coming.
4. *The simplicity and clarity of goals and priorities.* This clearly relates to the preceding point. The purpose of intro-ducing a nurse practitioner service should be to improve patient care. The clearer the goals and purpose, the more likely it is that all staff will have a shared understanding of the nurse practitioner project, and therefore the more likely it is to succeed.
5. *Co-operative inter-organization networks.* Departments within the Trust have to co-operate to make the nurse practitioner role work, while external organizations such as the Primary Care Trust and local GPs have to be fully involved in setting up the nurse practitioner project if they are to co-operate fully.
6. *Good managerial–clinical relations.* Middle managers interface with clinical work on a daily basis. Whatever the vision at senior level, middle managers must support nurse practitioners in their role if they are to be effective.
7. *Key people leading the change.* Introducing the nurse practitioner role will be easier if local opinion leaders such as senior consultants or the chief nurse together with middle managers give the idea their full support. These are important people to

target in the early stages of working the project up.

8. *Quality and coherence of the policy.* The project team must show how the quality of the nurse practitioner's work will be measured, and must also consider the effects of introducing the role on other aspects of health care if practice is to be coherent.

Our experience in working with and teaching hospital-based nurse practitioners confirms the importance of these factors. There has to be a coherent approach involving all the interested parties, and with a clear goal in mind. The nurse practitioner needs the support of a project team to ease the way forward, as changing practice is very stressful and the nurse practitioner cannot be left alone to carry through an organizational change that to many people is very radical, and at the same time develop a new, advanced clinical role. It is best to work initially with those areas of a hospital where the culture and context are most favourable to nurse practitioner role introduction. Demonstration of the success of the role strengthens the evidence base for change and will tend to weaken the fears that people may have, which are based upon the imagined implications of the role rather than the facts. If the context is not favourable, then the first task should be to improve it before attempting a nurse practitioner project. Approaching the problem the other way round is unlikely to succeed – i.e. introducing the nurse practitioner in the hope of improving the context as a result.

Relationships with other professional groups

As we have already seen, the nurse practitioner role is located on the boundary between medicine and nursing, and development of the role will be greatly facilitated by a co-operative dialogue with medicine. The negotiated order perspective (Reveley, 1999) indicates that the balance of power between nursing and medicine has to be renegotiated, ultimately for the patient's benefit, as nurse practitioners seek to expand their area of practice in such a way that they will begin to tread on medical territory. Reference was made in the intro-

ductory chapter to the need to avoid a turf war with medicine, and that theme will be developed throughout this book.

Walsh (2000) has advanced a simple analogy to deal with this issue. Imagine health care as a field of constant size with fixed boundaries. In this case, one group of practitioners can only expand their practice at the expense of another, and opposition to the nurse practitioner concept from medicine would be inevitable. However, the field of health care is more like the cosmological model of the expanding universe. It is growing bigger by the year as the population ages, new diseases appear, the social environment changes, technology makes more treatments possible, and new drugs come on the market to treat the previously untreatable. The whole field of health care in which nurse practitioners and medicine are located is expanding, and there is therefore ample space for nurses to expand their practice without threatening medicine. In fact, to stay with the cosmological analogy, failure to expand practice will only result in the appearance of black holes in the very fabric of that universe, black holes into which patients with unmet health care needs will disappear.

Some attempts to understand the growth of the nurse practitioner on the boundaries of nursing and medicine have fallen into the reductionist trap of trying to break medicine and nursing down into a simple list of tasks and then decide who does what. Cahill (1996) is guilty of such an approach, criticizing the nurse practitioner as focusing only on medical tasks. Barton *et al.* (1999) have a much more convincing argument when they point out that this is meaningless, as the labelling of tasks as medical or nursing is historically dated. There has been a movement of tasks between nursing and medicine ever since the emergence of modern health care, negating Cahill's criticisms. Blood pressure monitoring was once thought to be so difficult that only doctors could do it, whilst we now find some doctors learning counselling skills that nurses have used widely for many years. The approach of the UKCC in the *Scope of Professional Practice* document is all about getting away from lists of medical and nursing tasks. The emphasis instead is on looking at what needs to be done for the patient and ensuring that whoever carries out a task is competent to do so (UKCC, 1992). Barton *et al.* (1999) are correct to state that efforts which attempt to freeze boundaries by defining professions only in terms of skills lack insight into the very evolution of occupational groups and professions.

This point is taken further by Mitchell (1997), who argues that nurses who only define nursing in terms of a list of tasks should prepare themselves for replacement as they can be substituted by technicians who can be trained to carry out those tasks at a lower cost. Whether we are talking about nursing in general or the nurse practitioner role in particular, it is far more than a series of tasks. Those tasks have to be located in a matrix of ethical decision making and underpinned by knowledge to make coherent nursing practice. Registered nurses have to operate continually on feedback from the patient, and make decisions based on that feedback and on their knowledge base regarding what to do next. This ability to think on their feet and act with a high degree of autonomy and accountability is what differentiates nurses from technicians. Mitchell (1997) defines nursing in terms of quality, process and the meaningful experience of the patient rather than a list of tasks. To understand the role of nurses or nurse practitioners, it is necessary to look at what joins together the tasks they carry out. This is sometimes not obvious, especially to someone who is not a nurse, as the tasks are highly visible and easily recognized. The thought processes behind the motor skills, together with the use of psycho-social skills (giving support, utilizing active listening skills), are largely invisible.

The nurse practitioner role therefore is not about a series of tasks that nurse practitioners carry out but registered nurses in general do not. The tasks are the highly visible parts, but they are located within and connected together by a conceptual matrix consisting of clinical reasoning, ethical decision making, advanced knowledge and clinical experience of the role. Barton *et al.* (1999) argue for a fluid approach to the role as it is evolving in response to service need and in a cross-boundary environment. They speculate that nurse practitioners may be a new and discrete occupational group evolving out of nursing and medicine. Educational preparation for and evaluation of the role must therefore reflect this cross-boundary nature of the role. Finally they argue

that managers must give their nurse practitioner students full support if educationalists are to be able to prepare them fully for their nurse practitioner role.

Precisely this kind of task-oriented investigation of the nurse practitioner role has recently been carried out by Hicks and Hennessy (1999). Their study used a training needs analysis tool to show how the subject would see the nurse practitioner role and training needs. The authors state that the data this tool produces show how the respondents see the role relative to their own nursing role. As none of the nurses were nurse practitioners, it is questionable how much insight they had into the nurse practitioner role and therefore how much validity this kind of approach actually has. The sample was also rather unbalanced; 49 hospital clinical nurse specialists and 420 community nurses, with only a 22 per cent response rate amongst the primary care staff. This very low response rate again undermines the validity of this study, as systematic bias is an increasing risk with such low response rates. It may also indicate that as the primary care nurses were not working as nurse practitioners and had little insight into the role, they did not respond to the questionnaire, which again undermines the validity (and hence reliability) of the study. This research therefore has serious methodological and philosophical weaknesses.

These points have to be taken into account in interpreting the results claimed for this study. In their results, Hicks and Hennessy (1999) list a series of 11 role functions for the hospital nurse practitioner, which may be summarized as predominantly clinical examinations/diagnosis and research activity. Their data have statistically significant differences when comparing hospital with primary care nurses' view of the nurse practitioner role. Primary care nurses felt the following role functions were more important:

- Developing systems for patient recall
- Planning/conducting health promotion and other clinics
- Undertaking clinical examinations of patients
- Undertaking technical nursing procedures
- Using technical equipment.

Hospital staff felt that establishing relationships with patients and communicating with them face to face were more important aspects of the nurse practitioner role than did the primary care staff.

It is difficult to accept the claims made by the authors that this research demonstrates key differences between hospital and primary care nurse practitioner roles. Subjects in the study were each working with their own idea of what a nurse practitioner is, uncluttered by the experience of actually working with one. They defined the nurse practitioner role in terms of their own nursing role. The very low response rate further undermines the validity of this study. Perhaps the most that can be said for this research is that it demonstrates the confusion that surrounds the nurse practitioner role and the problems of working with task-oriented definitions. It certainly does not map out differences between hospital and primary care nurse practitioner roles with any reliability, especially given the small sample size of the hospital nurses involved.

Barton *et al* (1999) are more accurate when they state that nurse practitioners have a series of general skills that all registered nurses possess, to which they have added a new set of general skills that registered nurses do not have (history taking, physical examination, clinical decision making, differential diagnosis). Within the hospital setting, nurse practitioners practise these skills in a range of specialist departments such as accident and emergency, orthopaedics, urology and ear, nose and throat. The way they practise those skills – the invisible part of their work – is absolutely crucial to defining their work as nurse practitioners. If skills are part of the science of nursing, then joining them together into the process of care is where the art comes into play, whether it be as registered nurse or as nurse practitioner. Tasks are the bricks out of which we build walls, but a wall will not stand very long without mortar to bind it together. Investigations and definitions of the nurse practitioner role must look at the mortar as well as the bricks. The thought processes, knowledge, education and authority that the nurse practitioner possesses are as essential as sand, cement and water in mixing that mortar.

This analogy can be taken further, as the basic elements of bricks, stone and mortar can be assembled into many different buildings – some highly effective and functional, others

very beautiful, and some combining the best of both worlds. We also know the same ingredients can be combined to produce squalid buildings that do not serve any useful purpose at all. The difference between these various types of building is explained by factors such as careful planning, a design that is fit for purpose and function, spending the correct amount of money on the project, seeking the views of those who would use the building, and letting the architect use some imagination. The same principles clearly apply to developing the nurse practitioner role in hospital!

Legal issues and the nurse practitioner role

There is understandable concern about issues such as negligence and liability when introducing such a radical new role as the nurse practitioner. Nurse practitioners are wise to be cautious for, as Mark Twain once famously observed, it is better to be careful a hundred times than to be killed once! (Proehl, 2000). The legal implications of expanding nursing roles have been discussed by Walsh (2000), amongst others. In the limited space available here we will address the key issues that impact upon the nurse practitioner role.

This whole area is covered by common law (not the criminal justice system), which is sometimes called 'judge made' in that various judges have made rulings in the past on specific issues of principle and these have set precedents that are subsequently followed. Negligence was originally defined by a nineteenth century ruling that still stands today (Blyth *v* Birmingham Water Works 1891, cited in Young (1994), p. 24):

Negligence is the omission to do something which a reasonable man, guided upon these considerations which ordinarily regulate the conduct of human affairs would do, or to do something which a prudent and reasonable man would not do.

The phrase 'nurse practitioner' should be substituted for 'man' to translate this definition into modern clinical practice. Two key things are obvious from this ruling, the first of which is that if the nurse practitioner is not sure what to do, doing nothing is not an option! Omitting to do something can be negligence as much as doing the wrong thing. The second point is the key word 'reasonable'. The courts only expect nurse practitioners to be reasonable in their practice.

If a patient decides to bring a claim for compensation as a result of negligence by the nurse practitioner, the claim has to meet the following legal tests:

- That the defendant (nurse practitioner) owed the plaintiff (patient) a duty of care (in Scottish law, the term is pursuer rather than plaintiff). The very nature of the nurse practitioner–patient relationship ensures that this test will be met.
- That there was a breach in that duty of care.
- That breach led to harm to the patient which was not too distant in time from the original event. Harm therefore has to be demonstrated which is directly linked to a breach in the duty of care. If no harm occurred, it is not negligence in the legal sense of the term even though professionally the nurse practitioner may be judged to have acted unwisely or carelessly.
- The harm was a reasonably foreseeable consequence of that breach in the duty of care. An idiosyncratic drug reaction would not be foreseeable and therefore not negligence, but if the patient's notes had 'Allergic to penicillin', for example, written on the front in red, yet the nurse or nurse practitioner went ahead and gave penicillin, then that would clearly be foreseeable harm and consequently negligent.

At this point it is worth going back to the original 1891 definition of negligence to see if we can clarify what that rather vague word 'reasonable' actually means. Mr Justice McNair attempted to do just that in a case concerning Bolam *v* Friern Hospital Management Committee (1957), and his definition has become known as the Bolam test for reasonable practice (cited in McHale *et al.*, 1998, p. 19):

The test is the standard of the ordinary skilled man exercising and professing to have that specialist skill. A man need not possess the highest expert skill; it is well established law that it is sufficient if he exercises the ordinary skill of an ordinary competent man exercising that particular art.

This judgement was originally concerned with the practice of medicine. If we substitute 'nurse practitioner' for man, this throws up an interesting conundrum. It is quite clear that the Bolam test applies to a doctor. Are we therefore saying that the nurse practitioner has to achieve the standard of the ordinary skilled doctor, or the standard of the ordinary skilled nurse or nurse practitioner? If we look at this question from the patients' perspective the answer is obvious; they would expect the nurse practitioner to function at the standard of the ordinary skilled doctor if the procedure about to be undertaken was previously performed by a doctor.

A case heard in 1986 (Wilsher *v* Essex Area Health Authority) sheds light on this issue. The judge, Mr Justice Glidewell, stated that trainee doctors must be judged by the same standards as their more experienced colleagues, otherwise inexperience could be used as a defence against negligence claims. The message is clear; if you are not sure what you are doing, then you should not be doing it. Legal opinion confirms this point of view in relation to nursing and, although no court case has firmly established this precedent, Kloss (1988) states that the nurse who takes on roles that were once accepted as medical will be judged by the standard of a reasonable doctor. In hospital practice, therefore, the nurse practitioner has to be able to perform at the standard of a reasonable doctor when, for example, taking a medical history, carrying out a physical examination or ordering investigations such as radiography. Hence it would be prudent to ensure that the nurse practitioner has had educational preparation for the role at the same standard as a doctor, which is Honours degree level.

One final consideration is the concept of vicarious liability. In law, the employer has a responsibility for the actions of the employee, provided that the employee is not operating outside normal work practices and is not working for his or her own personal gain at the time of the incident. In practice this means that the plaintiff usually sues the employer for damages rather than the employee, as more compensation will be obtained via that route. The implications for the nurse practitioner are that, if things did go wrong, the Trust would be sued rather than the nurse practitioner, provided that the nurse practitioner was operating within his or her job description and not for personal gain. It is therefore always important to work within Trust guidelines and to ensure the Trust Board has approved any significant expansion in role.

Nurses are very familiar with the concept of consent, but this is an issue that should be revisited when setting up a new nurse practitioner service. Failure to obtain consent for any procedure could be deemed negligent, or could lead to a claim for damages on the grounds of the civil tort of assault and battery (a tort means a wrong in civil law). In effect, the nurse practitioner would have committed a trespass upon the person by touching the patient without consent. There is a difference between consent and informed consent, as the latter implies that the patient knows enough about what is happening to give a valid consent. If the patient does not realize that the person seeing them is not a doctor, consent cannot be valid as it is not informed consent. It is therefore absolutely essential that patients fully understand that they are being seen by a nurse practitioner, and the onus is on the nurse to make this clear. Failure to do so may lead to a claim for damages on the grounds that a procedure was carried out by a nurse when the patient thought the member of staff was a doctor. Even if no harm occurs, a claim for compensation upon the grounds of assault and battery may be pursued, as the nurse practitioner acted without the patient's informed consent.

Nurse practitioners and prescribing

No account of the hospital nurse practitioner role would be complete without considering the issue of prescribing. This term is used loosely by many nurses, and it is important to be precise about its legal meaning as opposed to the supply or administration of medicines. The Crown Report (1999) offers the following definitions of prescribing:

To order in writing the supply of a prescription-only medicine (POM) for a named patient.

To authorize by means of an NHS prescription the supply of any medicine, not just a POM, at public expense.

To advise a patient on suitable care or medication, including medicines which may be purchased over the counter. This definition is only used occasionally.

The only personnel who can legally write a prescription for a POM are doctors and dentists.

The term 'supply' is used in this context to mean providing a medicine to a patient or carer for administration. Doctors and dentists can supply medicines, but in the main this is carried out by pharmacists. However, a doctor or dentist can direct a nurse or other health professional to supply medicines in either a hospital or a health centre. Administration of a medicine simply means giving the medicine to the patient by whatever route is appropriate.

This legal framework greatly hinders the work of the nurse practitioner. It may be that having assessed the patient and arrived at a diagnosis the nurse practitioner is unable to proceed further with treatment for want of a prescription. The patient is then referred back to a doctor or kept waiting while the nurse practitioner seeks a medical signature on a prescription pad, either way wasting time and holding up treatment. The 1990s saw the development of group protocols as a way around this problem, and they were defined by the Crown Report (1998) as:

A specific written instruction for the supply and administration of named medicines in an identified clinical situation.

The protocol therefore applies to groups of patients, and not an individually named person. Ideally it should be drawn up locally by doctors and pharmacists after consultation with appropriate professional groups, and then approved by senior Trust management. The Crown Report (1998) was very critical of many of the group protocols it reviewed, and considered they fell well below acceptable safety standards. Doubts were also raised by some NHS unions about the legality of group protocols. The Crown Report felt there was a useful role for group protocols in facilitating care, and recommended that they must be drawn up in such a way that they are unambiguous, with clear lines of accountability and clinical criteria for use.

Nurse practitioners have used group protocols extensively in recent years, and have therefore been very concerned to ensure that they are legal, safe and effective. A positive step forward came in the summer of 2000, when amendments to the Medicines Act 1968 were passed into law and clarified the legal status of what are now known as patient group directions (PGDs). As a result, staff may legally supply and administer medicines to groups of patients who are not individually identified prior to treatment (Parish, 2000). The amendments also contain guidance on how PGDs should be drawn up, echoing the views of the Crown Report (1998) that a senior doctor and pharmacist must be involved and they must both sign the final document, whilst the Trust or Primary Care Group must authorize their use.

Nurse practitioners may therefore operate legally with PGDs, as they now should be called, which is a welcome step forward. However, the much bigger battle remains to be won, which is for prescribing rights for nurses. The Crown Report (1999) addressed this issue, and recommended that prescribing rights be extended to other health professionals in certain circumstances. Two categories of prescriber were suggested; independent and dependent prescribers. The former would be able to prescribe medicines, after carrying out a thorough assessment, as part of their patient management, while the latter would be able to vary prescriptions already written within an agreed treatment plan. Nurse practitioners would clearly fit the independent prescriber description, and implementation of the Crown Report (1999) would be a real quantum leap forward for them. Discussions are under way at the Department of Health (DoH, 2000) at present regarding this report, with much debate centring on what sort of formulary nurses would have access to. The simple approach would be to let nurses have access to the entire *British National Formulary* and rely upon the *Scope of Professional Practice* (UKCC, 1992) document to regulate the way nurses that utilize the formulary. Alternative suggestions envisage a series of different formularies depending upon the clinical area that the nurse practices in. This could lead to a bureaucratic nightmare, as nurses cover so many different specialities that we could end up with 20–30 different nursing formularies. The RCN are pursuing this issue with the government at present, and by the time this book comes to print we might have had a clear and positive outcome from these discussions.

References

Barton, T., Thorne, R. and Hoptroff, M. (1999). The nurse practitioner: redefining occupational boundaries? *Int. J. Nursing Studies*, **36**, 57–63.

Bold, A. (1985). June 1967 at Buchenwald. In: *British Poetry Since 1945* (E. Lucie-Smith, ed.). Penguin.

Cahill, H. (1996). Role definition: nurse practitioners or clinician's assistants? *Br. J. Nursing*, **5(22)**, 1382–6.

Coopers and Lybrand (1996). *Nurse Practitioner Evaluation Summary*. Coopers and Lybrand Health Practice.

Crown Report (1998). *Review of Prescribing, Supply and Administration of Medicines: A report on the Supply and Administration of Medicines under Group Protocols*. Department of Health

Crown Report. (1999). *Review of the Prescribing, Supply and Administration of Medicines*. Department of Health.

Curtin, M. and Lubkin, I. (1998). What is chronicity? In: *Chronic Illness, Impact and Interventions* (I. Lubkin and P. Larsen, eds), Jones and Bartlett.

Davies, C. (1996). Cloaked in a tattered illusion. *Nursing Times*, **92(45)**, 44–6.

Department of Health (2000). *The NHS Plan: A Plan for Investment, A Plan for Reform*, Cm. 4818 1. HMSO.

Hancock, C. (2000). Opening conference address. *Emergency Nursing 2000 and Beyond*, Heriot-Watt University, Edinburgh.

Hicks, C. and Hennessy, D. (1999). A task-based approach to defining the role of the nurse practitioner: the views of UK acute and primary sector nurses. *J. Adv. Nursing*, **29(3)**, 666–73.

Hunter, A. (2000). In with the new. *Health Service J.*, **3 August**, 16–17.

Kingdon, J. (1995). *Agendas, Alternatives and Public Policies*, 2nd edn. Harper Collins.

Kitson, A., Harvey, G. and McCormack, B. (1998). Enabling the implementation of evidence based practice: a conceptual framework. *Qual. Health Care*, **7**, 149–58.

Kloss, D. (1988). Demarcation in medical practice; the extended role of the nurse. *Professional Negligence*, **4(2)**, 41–7.

La Monica, E. (1990). *Management in Health Care*. Springers.

Lewin, K. (1951). *Field Theory in Social Sciences*. Harper and Row.

McHale, J., Tingle, J. and Peysner, J. (1998). *Law and Nursing*. Butterworth-Heinemann.

Mitchell, G. (1997). Re-engineering health care: why nurses matter. *Nursing Sci. Q.*, **10(2)**, 71.

Nursing Standard (2000). Health visitors left out of council's title. *Nursing Standard*, **14(47)**, 5.

Parrish, C. (2000). Supplying drugs under protocol is legal at last. *Nursing Standard.* **14(48),** 5.

Peterson, A. and Bunton, R. (1997). *Foucault; Health and Medicine.* Routledge.

Pettigrew, A., Ferlie, E. and McKee, L. (1992). *Shaping Strategic Change.* Sage.

Proehl, J. (2000). Respice, prospice: looking forward, looking back. Address to the Emergency Nursing 2000 and Beyond International Conference, Edinburgh.

Rapp, M. (2000). Advanced practice nursing in the postacute continuum for the older person. In: *Advanced Practice Nursing,* 2nd edn (J. Hickey, R. Ouimette and S. Venegoni, eds), Lippincott.

Reveley, S. (1999). Working with others; the nurse practitioner and role boundaries in primary health care. In: *Nurse Practitioners; Clinical Skills and Professional Issues* (M. Walsh, A. Crumbie and S. Reveley, eds), pp. 284–92. Butterworth-Heinemann.

Strauss, A., Schatzman, L., Ehrlich, D. *et al.* (1963). The hospital and its negotiated order. In: *The Hospital in Modern Society* (M. Freidson, ed.), Free Press.

Svensson, R. (1996). The interplay between doctors and nurses – a negotiated order perspective. *Sociology Health Illness,* **18(3),** 379–98.

United Kingdom Central Council for Nursing, Midwifery and Health Visiting (1992) *Scope of Professional Practice.* UKCC.

Walsh, M. (2000). *Nursing Frontiers; Accountability and the Boundaries of Care.* Butterworth-Heinemann.

Wilkinson, G. and Miers, M. (1999). *Power and Nursing Practice.* Macmillan.

Wong, S. (1999). Reimbursement to advanced practice nurses (APNs) through Medicare. *Image: J. Nursing Scholarship,* **31(2),** 167–73.

Young, A. (1994). *Law and Professional Conduct in Nursing.* Scutari.

3

CLINICAL NURSE SPECIALISTS, NURSE PRACTITIONERS AND LEVELS OF PRACTICE: WHAT DOES IT ALL MEAN?

Shirley Reveley

Introduction

This chapter provides an overview of some of the debates surrounding the roles of the clinical nurse specialist and the nurse practitioner. Where do the two types of role differ? What are the similarities? The plethora of nursing specialisms and titles means that the nursing profession itself is confused, let alone commissioners of health care and patients. Stilwell found that in one hospital alone there were over 50 specialist nurse titles (Stilwell, 1996), and Walsh reported over 40 nurse specialist titles in one Regional Health Authority (Walsh, 1996). A Department of Health funded study undertaken between 1995 and 1998, *Exploring New Roles in Practice* (ENRiP), entered 838 roles in its database (DoH, 1998). Of these, 603 (72 per cent) were nursing roles that were thought to be innovative and 235 (28 per cent) were for Professions Allied to Medicine. Nurses' titles included 'clinical nurse specialist', 'nurse practitioner', 'sister' or 'nurse', and some did not have the word nurse in the title at all (Levenson and Vaughan, 1999).

The chapter also attempts to address the concept of advanced and specialist nursing practice. What do these terms mean? How does advanced nursing practice differ from specialist nursing practice? Can the research undertaken help us clarify the issues, or will advanced nursing practice always remain an enigma (Woods, 2000)?

First, a brief overview of nurse practitioner and clinical nurse specialist roles is given.

Nurse practitioners

The nurse practitioner role has been the subject of considerable British research (Stilwell *et al.*, 1987; Salisbury and Tettersell, 1988; Chambers, 1994; Greenhalgh and Co.

Ltd, 1994; Read and Graves, 1994; Marsh and Dawes, 1995; Poulton, 1995; Cash and Hannis, 1996; Reveley, 1999). Despite the increasing amount of British research, coupled with the vast amount from the USA, there is still no consensus on how to define the nurse practitioner role in the United Kingdom. However, at St Martin's College our view of nurse practitioner practice is in line with the views expressed by a group of nurse practitioner educators who gave evidence to the UKCC in 1998. This states that nurse practitioners should:

- Reflect upon, articulate and operationalize their own philosophy of care
- Critically assess health care demands and act as a catalyst for innovations that meet the needs of their clients through the considered use of evidence-based practice
- Offer direct care to patients and families
- Possess enhanced consultation skills, including the ability to conduct a comprehensive, holistic assessment and clinical examination, working across usual nursing boundaries
- Make professionally autonomous decisions for which they have sole responsibility
- Act as referral agents and co-ordinators of care
- Have the knowledge and skills to assess and manage patients with a wide range of health problems, which includes medical diagnosis
- Have prescribing rights.

Watson *et al.* (1994. p. 4) state that:

A significant amount of what has been written comes from advocates or pioneers of the role ... and much has been made of the work of a small number of individual practitioners. Moreover, they suggest that the literature tends to be descriptive, journalistic and promotional.

Since 1994, however, two major evaluation studies have been undertaken (Touche Ross,

1994; Coopers and Lybrand, 1996). In addition, Reveley (1999) undertook a longitudinal study into the role of the nurse practitioner in general practice. These studies add much weight to the small-scale studies cited above.

Much of the early research was undertaken by practitioners reflecting on their role; many commentators attempted to define what the role actually entailed. These attempts to describe the nurse practitioner role usually produced lists of attributes or characteristics that emphasize the unique aspects of the role, such as the acquisition of assessment and diagnostic skills, and also emphasized the holistic nature of nurse practitioner practice. Perhaps the most widely quoted example of what the role entails is provided by Bliss and Cohen (1977; see p. 7), who say that the first official definition of the nurse practitioner role came from the American Nurses Association (ANA) in 1974. This definition was linked to statements concerning the educational needs of nurses with an expanded scope of practice.

Bowling and Stilwell (1988) argue that it is not just a range of tasks, or diagnosis and treatment skills, that define the work of the nurse practitioner. Rather they contend that these skills are integral to the role, but the nurse practitioner role also represents a philosophy of autonomous nursing practice and accountability for that practice.

Watson *et al.* (1994) expressed doubts as to the usefulness of lists as a means of classification. They suggest that such lists refer to 'organisational and structural factors, to the activities and processes of work in addition to occupational ideologies and boundaries'. Defining the nurse practitioner role should focus on the thinking and decision making that makes the nurse practitioner different from the conventional nurse, and also look at the patient's perception of the nurse practitioner. Seeing the patient as the first point of contact and functioning with a much greater degree of autonomy than usual in nursing does lead the nurse practitioner to think in qualitatively different ways. Bringing together the history and examination findings to arrive at a working diagnosis and then managing the uncertainty inherent in that process are new skills that traditional nursing has not embraced. Being a nurse practitioner is about working with probabilities and managing risk in a way unfamiliar to many nurses. As nurses develop

into the nurse practitioner role, they frequently say this is the biggest change they have noticed. Above all, research findings consistently demonstrate that patients appreciate the new role. Mitchell's two tests of what constitutes nursing can therefore be applied to defining the nurse practitioner role.

Statements about the attributes of the nurse practitioner are also sometimes unhelpful in that they often use various terms interchangeably without offering clarification. For example, 'advanced practice' is a relative term. This can mean advanced relative to a newly qualified nurse, a nurse of 2 years' standing or a first-year student. It only makes sense if there is a benchmark of practice that the 'advanced' term refers to. The term 'autonomous practice' has been extensively analysed by Walsh (2000), who argues that the term autonomous means different things when applied to nursing collectively or the individual nurse. Further, nobody is actually totally autonomous in the National Health Service; even the most senior surgeons cannot do whatever they like independently of anybody else! Autonomy is therefore a relative term, and should be used as such. Other phrases used in connection with the nurse practitioner are 'accountability for practice' and 'an expanded nursing role', both of which apply to all registered nurses, not only to nurse practitioners.

The nurse practitioner movement in the UK has developed at a time of much change in health care and upheaval for nursing, and is still in its infancy. It would therefore be very surprising to find the role neatly defined with all the loose ends tied up. It is an evolving and developing role, which makes it an exciting area in which to work and gives us a great deal of freedom. Uncertainty is sometimes the price that has to be paid for opportunity.

The clinical nurse specialist–nurse practitioner relationship

The development of the clinical nurse specialist role in the USA began in the 1960s, and was intended to improve quality of care for patients and to keep expert nurses with specialized skills at the bedside, the only other options for advancement being education or management (Parrinello, 1997). In the UK the development of clinical nurse specialists began in the 1970s, and the Joint Board of Clinical Nursing Studies provided a range of post-registration courses. These tended to follow medical specialities (Castledine, 1998). The development of the clinical nurse specialist role in the UK also encouraged nurses to remain 'at the bedside'. Castledine (1998) provides a useful overview of early nurse specialist roles in the UK.

Read and Graves (1994) stated that the level of practice for both clinical nurse specialists and nurse practitioners is advanced, and that these two nursing roles have developed simultaneously over the past 20 years in the UK. The 'specialist' component of the clinical nurse specialist title is generally seen to come from a specialist area of practice derived from the clinical specialities of medicine – for example, diabetes nurse specialists, rheumatology nurse specialists and many more. This assumes that each specialist area of nursing practice has its own body of knowledge and skills. It is perfectly possible for a clinical nurse specialist to display all the characteristics of a nurse practitioner; however, the role is defined and works within a specialist area. Within hospitals, for example, it is possible to have such a role as a specialist nurse practitioner. Watson *et al.* (1994) agree, pointing out that some nurse practitioners' work is difficult to distinguish from that of the nurse specialist, which leads to the question of 'what's in a name anyway?'.

The United Kingdom Central Council for Nursing, Midwifery and Health Visiting (UKCC) argued that there was a fundamental difference between being engaged in advanced practice and simply working in a speciality (UKCC, 1994). This conceptual confusion on the part of the UKCC seriously hindered the introduction of their Post-Registration Education for Practice (PREP) programme. After several years they finally had to abandon what had become an untenable position and dispense with the use of the term 'specialist' to describe a level of practice. The term 'specialist' only defines a field of practice, within which a nurse could be a complete novice (e.g. the first day as a staff nurse on intensive care), competent, proficient, or an expert. Only those nurses who have advanced their knowledge and skills through education and experience can exercise increasing clinical

discretion and accept greater responsibility through advanced practice. The generally held view of the specialist nurse as one who has specific expertise related to a particular area of clinical practice therefore did not accord with the UKCC's view of specialist practice as being a level of practice.

Barton *et al.* (1999) suggest that a specialist '… is commonly associated with an individual who focuses on a particular practical or theoretical branch of their profession'. They argue that the nurse practitioner role is a generalist one in that nurse practitioners have particular skills that are transferable, allowing them to practice in a wide range of clinical settings. They further argue that the generic skills of a nurse practitioner extend beyond those usually associated with nursing or medicine, making it a unique role. Nurse practitioners have highly developed skills of physical assessment, diagnosis, treatment and prescribing which sets them apart from other nurses, and many commentators see this as at the level of an advanced practitioner. These portable skills which help to define the nurse practitioner role have to be allied with an in-depth knowledge of a particular clinical area and group of patients (clinical speciality) in order to allow the nurse practitioner to become a specialist nurse practitioner in, for example, urology, accident and emergency or orthopaedics. If, however, advanced practice is seen slightly differently, as one in which the nurse acts as researcher, manager and innovator, pushing back the boundaries of nursing, then not all nurse practitioners would fit the description of advanced practitioner. Many nurse practitioners are practising advanced clinical skills that extend into the medical domain, and it is this aspect of the role that blurs the medical/nursing boundary and gives rise to confusion about advanced and specialist practice. This raises the issue as to whether a particular nurse practitioner is an advanced nurse or a substitute doctor. Most research reports have avoided discussion of this, but it is an important consideration. According to Emmerson (1996), the nurse practitioner is a role that is complementary to that of medicine, which 'increases patient choice, adds diversity to patient care, enhances collaboration with the medical profession and enhances the scope of the skill mix across the [primary] health-care team'.

So what are the differences, if any, between clinical nurse specialists and nurse practitioners? Clinical nurse specialists focus on education, clinical research, system improvement and outcomes management. Parrinello (1997) explains that the clinical nurse specialist role in the USA has 'a primary focus on the health care system and patient care from an aggregate perspective. The provision of direct care to patients and families is typically the secondary focus of the clinical nurse specialist role'. For the nurse practitioner it is the reverse, the primary focus being the patient, with systems being secondary. Thus:

Nurse practitioner

- Direct patient care including physical and psychosocial assessment, health history, diagnosis, treatment.

Clinical nurse specialist

- Education
- Clinical research
- System improvement
- Outcomes management.

Shah (1997, p. 102), another American writer, explains the difference as follows:

Although some areas of interest, such as education or patient care, are identical, the spheres of influence are different. The Advanced Nurse Practitioner (ACNP) is responsible for the patient plan of care. This could involve planned or spontaneous educational sessions with other nurses. The Clinical Nurse Specialist (CNS), on the other hand, may be responsible for the overall level of clinical expertise of the staff on a particular unit. The ACNP provides consultation in numerous patient situations with many of the staff. The CNS provides consultation for the entire unit by representing it on various hospital committees and other forums.

This position could be simply summarized by saying that the advanced nurse practitioner is directly involved in hands-on care, while the clinical nurse specialist is more concerned with policy and unit management. These lines of demarcation are not so clear-cut in the UK; nurse practitioners also act as consultants to other nurses on the unit, and clinical nurse specialists provide direct patient care. Shah's distinction then is not really helpful to us. Is it

time to merge the roles of nurse practitioner and clinical nurse specialist? Certainly in the USA there is much debate about this, and since 1996 there has been a gradual coming together of the roles. This has also been driven by economic factors, as hospitals have perceived the advanced nurse practitioners as offering better value for money with their hands-on care than the clinical nurse specialists. We have argued elsewhere (Reveley and Walsh, 2000) that educational programmes for nurse practitioners in primary care and community specialist practitioners could come together in an overarching framework. This framework could also be adapted to provide an integrated educational programme for hospital nurse practitioners and clinical nurse specialists in secondary care. Cronenwett (1995) argues that all segments of the nursing profession need to work together towards a common goal so that the advanced practice nurse can fulfil a variety of roles. The arguments for and against merging the roles have been summarized as follows (Soehren and Schumann, 1994, cited in Cronenwett, 1995, p. 112).

FOR:

- Many similarities already exist in these roles
- Practice settings for both are expanding and overlapping
- Unity and an increase in numbers would give more power to advanced practitioners
- Many similarities already exist in educational preparation
- Increased cost-effectiveness for colleagues and universities would result if programmes were combined
- Graduates with both qualifications would be more marketable.

AGAINST:

- Scope of practice remains different; typically nurse practitioners are generalists in managing illness and promoting health and clinical nurse specialists are acute care sub-specialists
- Legal entanglements exist as the nurse practitioner qualification in the UK is not recordable on the UKCC Register
- Problems arise with titles regarding name recognition and legal issues
- There may be lengthening of education programmes leading to recruitment problems.

Page and Arena (1994, p. 117) point out that if the two roles are merged in the USA it will result in role blurring and confusion, and too much role strain for practitioners. In addition, nurses in merged roles might find it hard to retain a nursing focus rather than a medical focus and thus the profession will be jeopardized. In a 1995 article Cronenwitt addresses all these issues and concludes that:

The walls that divide inpatient, outpatient, primary, tertiary and community care are coming down and society should expect that the nursing profession will prepare and regulate advanced nursing practice for the good of patient care and society as a whole. To do so schools with clinical graduate programmes must create a consistent product; credentialling (statutory) bodies must use consistent criteria to acknowledge advanced practice knowledge and expertise, and (state boards of) nursing must give legal recognition for advanced practice to these same nurses.

This statement appears sensible, but is it achievable? Certainly in the USA, which is where Cronenwitt is writing, the merging of the nurse practitioner and clinical nurse specialist roles is still under debate. However, consistent features of preparation for advanced nursing practice in the USA seem to be that it is at Masters level (which is not necessarily the same as Masters level in the UK), and that advanced practice as a concept seems to be accepted. However, Cronenwett (1995) tells us that the distinction between specialist and advanced nursing practice is not really clear-cut. She tells us that, in the 1980s, the ANA credentialling bodies and the nursing speciality organizations 'were certifying nurses at the generalist level for the specialty practice they had acquired through continuing education and experience'. So what is the distinguishing feature of specialist practice if it occurs in both generalist and specialist nursing practice? To complicate matters further, the public and nursing bodies were increasingly using the term 'advanced practice', and it was not clear whether this had a different meaning from specialist practice. These debates also abound in the UK nursing literature, and the UKCC set up working groups in the late 1990s to look at this very issue.

Advanced and specialist nursing practice

In a 1994 document, the UKCC established specialist practice as a higher level of practice than that required for initial registration. This document, *Standards for Education and Practice Following Registration* (UKCC, 1994), stated that those practitioners with a first degree in their area of practice are specialist practitioners, and that there is another level of nursing practice that constitutes advanced practice:

Advanced nursing practice is concerned with adjusting the boundaries for the development of future practice, pioneering and developing new roles responsive to changing needs and, with advancing clinical practice, research and education to enrich professional practice as a whole.

However, there was no statement about how nurses may become registered as advanced practitioners, and standards for education and practice for advanced practitioners were not elucidated. Rather, there was an intimation that advanced practice would be at Masters level, and that the profession itself would decide how advanced practice was to be defined. Advanced practice was seen as that sphere of professional practice concerned with continuing professional development, for which some practitioners would wish to gain additional skills and knowledge up to Masters degree level. These statements led immediately to a hierarchy of practice that was interpreted by most people as initial, specialist and advanced practice. Many Masters courses were developed in universities, and even though the UKCC stated that a hierarchy of levels of practice was not intended, that is exactly what happened.

What also happened was that there was (and is) confusion regarding the term 'specialist practice' in relation to whether it is seen as a level of practice or an area of clinical expertise that is concerned with a particular client group. In Read and Roberts-Davis's (2000) Delphi study, the nurses interviewed saw nurse practitioners as generalists dealing with a wide range of undifferentiated conditions, whilst clinical nurse specialists were seen as specialists dealing with a specific condition or client group. The nurse practitioner role was seen as 'specialist plus', in that something in addition to specialist practice was required for the role.

The Delphi study cited above demonstrated that there is considerable overlap in nurse practitioner and clinical nurse specialist roles.

Both share nursing competencies, and many clinical nurse specialists may be expanding their practice such that they need to take on the same competencies as nurse practitioners. Experience of teaching both nurse practitioners and clinical nurse specialists over a number of years leads us to agree with this and to question how much longer we should go on educating these two groups of nurses separately.

The Delphi study also showed that the difference between clinical nurse specialist and nurse practitioner roles lies in the focus of their practice and the patient conditions that each deals with. The clinical nurse specialist works with a specific client group, often over a long period of time, and the condition has been diagnosed before the patient comes into the clinical nurse specialist's care. Nurse practitioners, on the other hand, are generalists seeing a wide range of undifferentiated conditions, and the interaction with the patient may be for a short time or for short recurrent periods. This finding is not surprising, as it stems from seeing nurse practitioners as only working in primary health care, where the generalist role is paramount. It shows the importance of careful definition of terms and of context. Hospital nurse practitioners work in a different context to primary care nurse practitioners, and consequently will have a different client group to which they apply the same defining principles of care that differentiate nurse practitioners from conventional registered nurses. The result is that there are significant differences as well as commonalities in care.

We present evidence later of the importance of context in understanding nurse practitioner roles. For example, Chapters 5 and 6 in this volume describe how two nurse practitioners are working with a specific client group who come to the nurse practitioner with diagnosed conditions (surgical or orthopaedic); thus these nurses could be said to be clinical nurse specialists. However, both are working in pre-operative assessment clinics and are assessing patients holistically to see if they are fit for surgery. This assessment goes beyond screening in that the nurses are using their own clinical judgement as to whether the patient can be admitted for surgery, needs referring for investigations or should have surgery deferred because there is some undiagnosed condition that requires treatment. Furthermore, these nurse practitioners are seeing the patients for longer periods of time as they develop pre-assessment advice and education and post-operative follow-up services. Thus they are developing relationships with the patient and carers over a longer period than that suggested in the Delphi survey.

A further difference between the two roles relates to legal and ethical issues (Read and Roberts-Davis, 2000). There is ambiguity about the legal and professional status of nurse practitioner roles, whereas clinical nurse specialist roles are recognized by the UKCC. For example, there are one Registerable and seven Recordable qualifications in community nursing specialist practice. The legal position of the nurse practitioner in the UK is discussed by Walsh in Chapter 2 of this volume.

It is difficult to apply the term 'advanced' to nursing nowadays, because in 1997 the UKCC stated that standards would not be set for advanced practice. 'Advancing' practice, where nursing practice is moved on in a dynamic and autonomous way, would be accepted, but it was the existing standards for specialist practice that would be the focus (Read and Roberts-Davis, 2000). In 1998 the UKCC tried to establish 'specialist' as a level of practice but, because there was found to be much confusion among employers, the nursing profession and the public, the title specialist practitioner is viewed as inappropriate and problematic.

The concept of advanced nursing practice then is highly contentious, and this has direct implications for the role and education of nurse practitioners, who practise an advanced nursing role. Although the literature on nurse practitioners sees their role as being an advanced nursing role, other nursing roles are also described as 'advanced', including that of the clinical nurse specialist. Sparacino and Durand (1986) stated that the advanced practitioner must:

- Portray sophisticated use of clinical knowledge
- Demonstrate high levels of accountability
- Carry out systematic assessment and intervention
- Demonstrate independent clinical decision making
- Participate in risk taking

- Portray autonomy and independence
- Expand the boundaries of nursing practice.

Mitchinson (1996, p. 34) defines advanced practice as:

Professional practice which is negotiated and developed by individual practitioners who are solely responsible and accountable to the patient and their professional body for their actions and omissions.

She draws a distinction between advanced practice and independent practice by stating:

Independent practice can be defined as practice which is assigned to and developed by individual practitioners who are then responsible and accountable for their actions which are undertaken without direct supervision or monitoring from any other practitioner or manager.

Castledine (1991, p. 34) stated that many of the skills of the advanced practitioner appear very similar to those used in the practice of medicine. He suggests, however, that:

The advanced practitioner will be able to explore the differences and significance of nursing as opposed to medical techniques. Not only will physical assessment be used, but psychosocial assessment and advanced counselling skills will also be crucial.

It is helpful therefore to think of advanced practice as defined by these various authors as being a necessary but not sufficient condition for the nurse practitioner role. In other words, operating at a level that is well beyond a newly qualified registered nurse is necessary to be a nurse practitioner, but on its own is not sufficient for the nurse practitioner role. As a logical deduction from that statement, we can say that it is possible to be an advanced practitioner but not a nurse practitioner.

'Advanced practice', as described by many authorities, is perceived to be about autonomy, decision making, moving practice forward and the possession of sophisticated knowledge. These definitions are different from the UKCC's use of the term 'advanced practice', but they closely resemble the UKCC's definition of 'specialist practice'. The UKCC sees this 'specialist practice' as a level of practice beyond initial registration, and that preparation for such roles is at first degree level.

Higher level of practice and consultant nurses

In the summer of 1998 the UKCC issued a consultation document entitled *A Higher Level of Practice*, which outlined plans for a number of nurses to practise at a higher level. Successful individuals would have the suffix 'H' added to their name on the Professional Register. *The Higher Level of Practice* (HLP) project follows on from the 1994 *Post-Registration Education and Practice* project (PREP). It is aimed at the further regulation of nurses, midwives and health visitors who are working at levels beyond initial registration. A standard for HLP is needed to protect consumers through clarification for all stakeholders of what constitutes acceptable levels of competence for nurses working beyond initial registration standards. The box below shows the practice areas under which the nurse has to achieve the UKCC standard in order to be working beyond initial registration standards. The HLP standard makes it clear that Higher Level Practice relates to a level of practice rather than roles.

The word 'advanced' is deliberately omitted from the HLP discussion document, and the terms 'nurse practitioner' and 'clinical nurse specialist' are not protected. The UKCC did not indicate specific training programmes or define standards for these roles. It remains to be seen what the profession will decide regarding the Higher Level Practice, but it leaves nurse practitioners in the same position they were before, that is, with no prescribed training programme and no protected title.

Practice areas for a higher level of practice (adapted from UKCC, 1999)

Nurses, midwives and health visitors who are working at a higher level of practice develop health care knowledge and practice for health gain through:

- providing effective health care
- improving quality and health outcomes
- evaluation and research
- leading and developing practice
- innovation and changing practice
- developing self and others working across professional and organizational boundaries.

Nurse practitioners wishing to be recognized as higher level practitioners will have to be assessed against national criteria, and these criteria will also apply to nurses in other roles who are expanding their practice. This is to provide regulation and standardization in practice. As this book goes to press, many nurse practitioners are in the process of trying to obtain recognition as higher level practitioners.

We believe that the BSc (Hons) Nurse Practitioner programme prepares nurses with those competencies required for Higher Level Practice and so sets them on the way to achieving HLP. Nurse practitioners must, however, remember to use their nursing skills as well as their newly acquired technical skills if they wish to be recognized as higher level practitioners (Read and Roberts-Davis, 2000).

To add to the confusion regarding nursing titles and levels of practice, in September 1998 the Prime Minister announced that some nurses (unspecified) would bear the title 'consultant'. Advanced practice and the position of nurse practitioners was once again passed over without discussion. It is interesting to note that the concept of the nurse consultant was mentioned in the Briggs Report (DHSS, 1972). A Royal College of Nursing annual congress motion was carried in 1971 with the following wording (cited in Castledine and McGee, 1998, p. 19):

That this meeting of the RCN Representative Body strongly supports the recommendations in the RCN evidence to the Committee on Nursing that an advanced clinical role for the nurse/midwife be identified by the creation of posts of nurse/midwife consultant.

The title 'nurse consultant' adds to the number of titles nurses can hold and contributes to the confusion that patients have to deal with regarding roles. Furthermore, what does the title 'consultant' actually mean, and how does the role relate to consultant doctors? Will patients know the difference? Only time will tell, but the question of nurse practitioner status is once more thrown into the debating arena. In the document *Agenda for Change: Modernising the NHS Pay System* (DoH, 1999a), three grades of nurse were described; entry level, mid-level with several pay points, and the expert practitioner level. It was interpreted that the nurse consultant

---

Characteristics of higher level practice
(adapted from UKCC, 1999)

The higher level practitioners:

- spend most of their time in direct patient care
- understand the implications of the social, economic and political context of health care
- demonstrate deepening and widening of their knowledge and practice, and patients, clients and fellow professionals acknowledge their deeper knowledge and their enhanced skills
- use complex reasoning, critical thinking, reflection and analysis to inform their health assessments, clinical judgements and decisions
- assess and manage risk
- identify their own and others' personal development needs and take effective action to address them
- have a proven ability to develop practice
- take a lead in implementing health and social care policy, national frameworks and quality improvement
- develop innovative services and work across boundaries
- bring about change and development in their own and others' practice and within the services in which they work.

---

would come under the expert practitioner level. At the beginning of 2001 there is no agreement on these new pay scales, and the Pay Review Body in its December 2000 report declined to end the overlap between I grade and nurse consultant salaries, further exacerbating the confusion. The role of nurse consultant was also discussed in *Making a Difference* (DoH, 1999b, p. 35), where the role is described as 'expert practitioner'. This nurse will provide:

expert care ... clinical or public health leadership and consultancy to senior registered practitioners and others ... and initiating and leading significant practice, education and service development.

Where will nurse practitioners lie in relation to the nurse consultant role? According to Read and Roberts-Davis (2000, p. 186), it is probable that the nurse consultant will be educated to doctoral level but that this will be a clinical doctorate rather than a research one.

The nurse practitioner and consultant nurse role are not the same. Most nurse practitioners are focused on clinical practice. They may be involved in audit and research, and they may be involved in supervision of others and in teaching and some service development, but it can be argued that these are secondary to the clinical role. Thus, some nurse practitioners may well become nurse consultants but they would need to refocus. Read and Roberts-Davis (2000) placed nurse practitioners in the Senior Registered Practitioner category as outlined in *Making a Difference* (DoH, 1999b), and would encompass building on nursing skills, providing leadership to registered practitioners, clinical management and/or specialist care. Preparation for this role would normally be at Masters level, and the person would have undertaken additional specialist-specific qualifications (DoH, 1999b).

Conclusion

It is against this background that the nurse practitioner role is developing, and the changes described do have an effect on traditional role boundaries and on staff morale (Traynor, 1993). The positive view on current policy developments is that now more than ever there are opportunities opening up for nurses. The pessimistic view is that to introduce yet another nursing role into this unsettled scene creates even more uncertainty and rivalry among nurses, with a corresponding retreat into tribalism (Beattie, 1995), which may lead to more fragmentation within nursing. One thing is for sure, we should only use terms like 'advanced' when they have been correctly defined and contextualized, recognizing that advanced practice, however defined, is a necessary but not sufficient condition for the nurse practitioner role. Finally, there is nothing contradictory or problematical about the term 'specialist nurse practitioner' being used in the hospital setting or for an outreach worker from a hospital base. It simply means a nurse utilizing the well-known skills, cognitive processes and role functions of a nurse practitioner within a specialized field of care.

References

Barton, T. D., Thome, R. and Hoptroff, M. (1999). The nurse practitioner: redefining occupational boundaries? *Int. J. Nursing Studies*, **36**, 57–63.

Beattie, A. (1995). War and peace among the health tribes. In: *Interprofessional Relations in Health Care* (K. Soothill, L. Mackay and C. Webb, eds). Edward Arnold.

Bliss, A. and Cohen, E. (eds) (1977). *The New Health Professionals: Nurse Practitioners and Physician Assistants*. Aspen Publications.

Bowling, A. and Stilwell, B. (eds) (1988). *The Nurse in Family Practice: Practice Nurses and Nurse Practitioners in Primary Health Care*. Scutari Press.

Cash, K. and Hannis, D. (1996). *The Evaluation of Nurse Practitioners Funded under the Junior Doctors' Hours Initiative: The Durham Model*. University of Durham.

Castledine, G. (1991). The advanced nurse practitioner (Part Two). *Nursing Standard*, **5(44)**, 33–6.

Castledine, G. (1998). Clinical specialists in nursing in the UK: the early years. In: *Advanced and Specialist Nursing Practice* (G. Casteldine and P. McGee, eds). Blackwell Science.

Castledine, G. and McGee, P. (eds) (1998). *Advanced and Specialist Nursing Practice*, p. 19. Blackwell Science.

Chambers, N. (1994). *The Derbyshire Nurse Practitioner Project*. Derbyshire Family Health Services Authority.

Coopers and Lybrand (1996). *Nurse Practitioner Evaluation Project: Final Report*. NHS Executive.

Cronenwett, L. R. (1995). Molding the future of advanced practice nursing. *Nursing Outlook*, **43(3)**, 112–18.

Department of Health and Social Services (1972). *Report of the Committee on Nursing*. Chairman Professor Asa Briggs. Cmnb 5115. HMSO.

Department of Health (1998). *Exploring New Roles in Practice: Implications of Developments within the Clinical Team*. A study funded by the Department of Health's Human Resources and Effectiveness Initiative. DoH.

Department of Health (1999a). *Agenda for Change: Modernising the NHS Pay System*. DoH.

Department of Health (1999b). *Making a Difference*. DoH.

Emmerson, P. (1996). Are nurse practitioners merely substitute doctors? *Professional Nurse*, **11(5)**.

Greenhalgh and Company Limited (1994). *The Interface Between Junior Doctors and Nurses: A Research Study for the Department of Health*. Greenhalgh and Company.

Levenson, R. and Vaughan, B. (1999). *Developing New Roles in Practice: An Evidence-based Guide*. School of Health and Related Research (SCHARR), University of Sheffield.

Marsh, G. N. and Dawes, M. L. (1995). Establishing a minor illness nurse in a busy general practice. *Br. Med. J.*, **310**, 778–80.

Mitchinson, S. (1996). Are nurses independent and autonomous practitioners? *Nursing Standard*, **10(34)**, 34–8.

Page, N. E. and Arena, D. M. (1994). Rethinking the merger of the clinical nurse specialist and nurse practitioner roles. *Nursing Policy*, **26(4)**, 315–18.

Parrinello, K. M. (1997). An administrative perspective on the acute care nurse practitioner role. In: *The Acute Care Nurse Practitioner* (B. J. Daly, ed.), pp. 111–39. Springer Publishing.

Poulton, B. (1995). Keeping the customer satisfied. *Primary Health*, **5(4)**, 16–19.

Read, S. and Graves, K. (1994). *Reduction of Junior Doctors' Hours in the Trent Region: The Nursing Contribution*. Trent RHA/NHS Executive

Read, S. and Roberts-Davis, M. (2000). Preparing nurse practitioners for the 21st century. From the report: *Realising Specialist and Advanced Nursing Practice: Establishing the Parameters of, and Identifying the Competencies for 'Nurse Practitioner' Roles and Evaluating Programmes of Preparation (RSANP)*. University of Sheffield.

Reveley, S. (1999). Introducing the nurse practitioner into a group general medical practice: operational and theoretical perspectives on role. Unpublished PhD thesis, University of Lancaster.

Reveley, S. and Walsh, M. (2000). Preparation for advanced nursing roles. *Nursing Standard*, **14(31)**, 42–5.

Salisbury, C. J. and Tettersell, M. (1988). Comparison of the work of a nurse practitioner with that of a general practitioner. *J. R. Coll. GPs*, **38**, 314–16.

Shah, S. S. (1997). Acquiring clinical skills and integrating them into the practice setting. In: *The Acute Care Nurse Practitioner* (B. J. Daly, ed.), p. 102. Springer Publishing.

Soerhen, P. M. and Schumann, L. L. (1994). Enhanced role opportunities available to the CNS/nurse practitioner. *Clin. Nurse Specialist*, **8**, 173–7.

Sparacino, P. and Durand, B. (1986). Editorial on specialisation. *Advanced Nursing Practice Momentum*, **4(2)**, 2–3.

Stilwell, B. (1996). Chair's remarks. *Making a World of Difference: Nurse Practitioners, A Global Perspective*. Fourth International Conference and Exhibition on Nurse Practitioner Practice, Heriot-Watt University, August 22–24.

Stilwell, B., Greenfield, S., Drury, V. W. M. and Hull, F. M. (1987). A nurse practitioner in general practice: working style and pattern of consultations. *J. R. Coll. GPs*, **37**, 154–7.

Touche Ross (1994). *Evaluation of Nurse Practitioner Projects*. Touche Ross Management Consultants Ltd.

Traynor, M. (1993) Community nurses: a culture of uncertainty. *Nursing Standard*, **7(37)**, 38–40

United Kingdom Central Council for Nursing, Midwifery and Health Visiting (1994). *Standards for Education and Practice following Registration*. UKCC.

United Kingdom Central Council for Nursing, Midwifery and Health Visiting (1998). *A Higher Level of Practice*. Consultation document: The UKCC's proposals for recognising a higher level of practice within the post-registration regulatory framework. UKCC.

United Kingdom Central Council for Nursing, Midwifery and Health Visiting (1999). *A Higher Level of Practice: Draft Descriptor and Standard*. UKCC.

Walsh, M. (1996). Nurse Practitioner: To Be or Not To Be? Paper presented at a nurse practitioner study day, Lancaster: St Martin's College.

Walsh, M. (2000). *Nursing Frontiers; Accountability and the Boundaries of Care*. Butterworth-Heinemann.

Watson, P., Hendey, N. and Dingwall, R. (1994). *Role Extension/Expansion with Particular Reference to the Nurse Practitioner*. School of Social Studies, University of Nottingham.

Woods, L. P. (2000). *The Enigma of Advanced Nursing Practice*. Quay Books.

4

MEDICINE, NURSING AND JURISDICTION OVER PATIENT CARE

Shirley Reveley

Introduction

Nurse practitioners in the hospital setting have recently found a niche for themselves in modern health care. In many hospitals the role has been introduced in response to the government initiative to reduce junior doctors' hours (NHSME, 1991), and this has created space for nurse practitioners to take the initiative in patient care. Descriptions of the nurse practitioner role often emphasize the acquisition of that knowledge and skills that were formerly firmly located in the medical domain, and this has led to debates about 'turf' – that is, who does what within health care. The introduction of nurse practitioners into hospitals, then, has thrown into sharp relief the work of medicine and nursing, and patient care can be seen to be a contested area among the health professions (Reveley, 1999). A book such as this would therefore be incomplete if it failed to address the roles of doctors and nurses and how they compete with, or complement, one another.

This chapter will examine medicine and nursing as occupational roles, and will utilize the work of Abbott (1988) to explore the extent to which these roles are contested. The chapter will give a brief overview of some of the main traditional theories of role and professions. It will focus on the professions of medicine and nursing from the perspective of Abbott's concept of 'jurisdiction'. This serves to illuminate the social and cultural context within which the professional boundary between doctors and nurse practitioners is negotiated. The chapter also explores the concept of the 'new nursing' (Beardshaw and Robinson, 1990; Witz, 1994) in relation to nurse practitioners.

Sociological perspectives on role

In social life people are expected to behave in certain ways in particular situations, and this expected behaviour is a 'role'. Professional training socializes professionals into expected behaviours, and such socialization depends on the historical development, training and ideologies of the profession concerned. Socialization is a complex process involving the acquisition of attitudes, emotions, thoughts, values, skills, motivations, knowledge and social patterns appropriate to enable the individual to cope with the physical, cultural, and social environment of a given society. The concept of 'professional role' is important in that it provides a means of analysing ways in which individuals relate to one another in organizations.

Role theory provides a conceptual framework for studying the ways in which individuals and groups behave together. Concepts of role derive from one or other of two schools of thought in social theory: the functionalist approach or symbolic interactionism.

The functionalist approach (Durkheim, 1964; Parsons, 1951) assumes that roles are more or less fixed and have attached to them certain expectations and obligations. The functionalist perspective maintains that institutions arise in society because they meet a particular need for that society. Roles are viewed as facts that are transmitted from one generation to the next in the process of socialization. They serve as essential prerequisites of the social system. The functionalist approach to role implies some degree of commitment to norms, for, in order to cooperate successfully and on a regular basis, a high degree of predictability is necessary. Individuals internalize social norms and behave in fairly predictable ways. Role expectations are seen to be complementary – e.g. between nurse and patients – and are backed up by rules and rewards (formal sanctions) or approval/disapproval (informal sanctions). But what about the situation where there is a low degree of predictability, as is the case with the introduction of the nurse practitioner role? Conflicts might involve others in the role set, such as in situations where there is a lack of clear boundary lines about the definition of a particular job. There might be problems of status (who tells who what to do), or there might be lack of congruence between what is learned in training and what the job actually entails in practice.

Symbolic interactionism, unlike functionalism, sees people as skilled and creative actors. Whereas functionalists view social action as 'learned responses', interactionists argue that individuals engage in interactions with others and select certain roles for action which have more relevance for that individual than others. To be cohesive, groups depend on shared norms, ideas or ideologies. The emphasis in health care is currently on teamwork, which involves social relationships and implies co-operation. Individuals conform and co-operate for a variety of reasons, including internal motivation and external pressures. Co-operation may be contractual or open and diffuse, but in any case co-operation involves reciprocity and interdependence.

The nurse practitioner role is developing within organizations at various levels – the NHS, the group general practice, the hospital ward and so on – and therefore organization also needs to be taken into account. Medicine is a profession, and nursing is aspiring to become one. An overview of the theory of professions is therefore apposite at this juncture.

Sociological perspectives on professions

There is a wide literature on the sociology of the professions. Early writers in this field such as Carr-Saunders and Wilson (1933) and Durkheim (1964) saw professions as organized groups of experts who applied specialized knowledge to cases. Medicine is seen by some theorists as an 'ideal type' profession that consists of desirable elements or traits which provide a checklist for other occupations aspiring to professional status to emulate (Larkin, 1983). These elements include an organized system of training, formal entry requirements and a code of ethics, and such defining characteristics of a profession became central features in later definitions (Abbott, 1988). Other approaches to the study of professions are based on particular aspects such as the control of specialized knowledge, and some studies of professions have concentrated on professionalization as a collective strategy to enhance rewards and power of members (see, for example, Larson, 1977) through the creation of an occupational monopoly. Others have concentrated on the role of professionals in terms of their relationship to the state or elitist groups (capitalist agency approaches).

Parsons (1951), writing from a functionalist perspective, saw the profession of medicine as a 'set of social relations regulated according to criteria other than those of the market' (Davies, 1979a). The distinctive feature of this theory of professions is the centrality of the doctor/patient relationship. Doctors are seen to be motivated by a service-orientation, to be morally neutral, achieving and collectively oriented. Patients are seen as passive recipients of medical care. The doctor–patient relationship is a mutually satisfying one, in that each role has rights and responsibilities, and, if carried out according to the 'script', is functional and integrative. However, this view of professional and patient roles is an ideal type and came under criticism by writers who demonstrated that patients are not always passive and do not always comply unquestioningly with doctors' orders.

Szasz and Hollender (1956) argue that the doctor–patient relationship varies according to the nature of the particular medical problem and where the consultation takes place. Byrne and Long (1976) analysed a large number of taped consultations between doctors and patients, and found that there was a power continuum of doctor–patient communication, ranging from patient ascendancy to doctor ascendancy. However, doctor-centred communication was by far the most common mode of interaction. Thus there are problems with the structural functionalist role theory, in that it does not deal successfully with patient negotiations in the doctor–patient relationship. Nor does it deal well with entry and exit into new social roles, the problem being intensified with regard to medicine because it is difficult to agree on what constitutes illness (Hart, 1985).

According to Larkin (1983), trait and functionalist approaches to the study of professions are concerned with the question 'what is a profession?', whilst monopoly and capitalist agency are concerned with 'under what set of circumstances do people in an occupation attempt to turn it into a profession?'. This latter question derived from the work of Everett Hughes (Larkin, 1983), and shifted the emphasis from the trait approach to the study of professions. Attention has also been given to the extent to which one profession (medicine) influences the professionalization projects of related occupations (Larkin, 1983; Witz, 1992). Abbott's (1988) work does not ask what a profession is, or about the circumstances that promote professionalism; rather, his book is concerned with how professions create their work and how they are created by it. It also offers explanations for interprofessional conflict. It is then a departure from the 'ideal type' approach. For Abbott (1988, p. 318), a profession is at one and the same time:

A form of organization, a level of social deference, an association with knowledge, and a way of organizing personal careers.

Abbott's work explores the way in which occupational groups control knowledge and skill. One way is to emphasize technique, which the craft professions do, another is to control abstract knowledge.

The symbolic interactionist perspective highlights the fact that roles are made, not merely occupied, and that professionalism is a claim that has to be justified (Davies, 1979a). Several theorists have concentrated their work on the profession of medicine itself, whilst others have looked at allied occupations such as nursing and midwifery (Abel-Smith, 1975; Donnison, 1977; Gamarnikow, 1978). Nursing has been much studied in relation to whether or not it is a profession. Nurses are often portrayed as less knowledgeable than doctors and less professional, and Davies (1979a) says that nurses borrow prestige from the medical profession. The professionalization project of nursing (Beardshaw and Robinson, 1990; Witz, 1994) seeks out a body of knowledge separate to that

of medicine, professional autonomy, self-regulation and accountability, higher education, full student status for learners, and government by a code of conduct and a code of practice. According to trait theory, then, nursing is a profession. Abbott (1988), however, argues that although these characteristics have been seen as traditional hallmarks of professionalism, they are not the only things; other occupations also have these characteristics but are not deemed to be professions.

Critics of functionalism, such as Freidson (1970) and Johnson (1972), insist that professionalism is about power. Johnson argues that 'a profession is not an occupation but a means of controlling an occupation' (cited in Davies, 1979a). Johnson contends that the way was opened for professionalization to occur by an expanding middle class at the time of the industrial revolution. This new middle class's demand for health care promoted the conditions for professionalism in terms of practitioners' control over clients (Larkin, 1983). Doctors also carved out a position for themselves in the nineteenth century voluntary hospitals but, according to Davies (1979a), social rank was a key means to doing this, functional expertise being a very recent concept.

The increasing technical innovation and demand led to the need for skilled assistance for doctors, and so auxiliaries were employed. Such a division of labour supported the status and income of those controlling the market (Larkin, 1983). The expansion of paramedical groups supplementary to medicine marked a further medical division of labour and reinforced the monopoly of medicine. It must not be assumed, however, that paramedical groups depend on medicine without the reverse being true. Larkin (1983) points out that over time medicine may become dependent on paramedical professions such as physiotherapists. Larkin describes paramedical workers in terms of: 'those occupations, excluding doctors, that have sought to organize as "professions", or at least claimed this status'. Such a group would include nurses, who have been embarking on a professionalization project (Witz, 1992) for many years. Etzioni (1969, cited in Larkin, 1983) used the term 'semi-professional' for paramedical groups on the grounds that a classification that assumes the complexity of modern knowledge requires a division of labour between applied and theoretical workers.

Larkin (1983) uses the term 'occupational imperialism' to refer to occupations attempting to shape the division of labour to their own advantage by, for example, taking skills from others or delegating them so that status and control are secured. Abbott (1988) supports this viewpoint, arguing that professions compete by taking over each other's tasks – 'the foundations of interprofessional competition are laid in the very acts of professional work itself' – and that 'jurisdiction is a more or less exclusive claim; one profession's jurisdiction affects those of others'.

Abbott (1988) uses the term 'collegiate professionals' to refer to social workers and nurses. He contends that the degree of abstraction needed for a profession to survive varies with time and space. In regard to this he cites the work of Larson (1977), who argued that some professions developed in aristocratic societies, others in democracies, and some under corporate capitalism and bureaucracy.

During the latter half of the twentieth century a new approach, the division of labour approach, came to the fore. Davies (1979a) believed that this called for a new way of conceptualizing available work, and broadened the discussion into what is health and what is illness, what are the responses to these, who are to be counted as health workers, and how are they regarded? This was a move away from traditional views of the division of labour espoused by the founding fathers of sociology. Durkheim (1964), for example, saw the division of labour as a feature of societies to be understood in terms of the transition from mechanical to organic solidarity, and that it had an integrative function. Weber (1947) saw a bureaucratic division of labour as rational planning towards a collective organizational goal set by political means. Marx, on the other hand, viewed the division of labour as planned but coercive, working in the interests of the dominant group (owners of production) and serving to coerce the subordinate group (workers) (Davies, 1979a).

According to Abbott (1988), the problem with current theories of professions is that they concentrate on structure rather than work. The content of the work of professionals is changing, he contends, and the control of work brings professions into conflict with one another. In relation to medicine and nurse practitioners, conflict can arise regarding both the content (more doctoring, less nursing) and the control of the nurse practitioner's work (the quest for more autonomy). Outside bureaucratic organizations (for example, in their work with homeless people), nurse practitioners have a far greater degree of control over their work than they do in hospital, where consultants have the final say and can supervise the nurse practitioner.

The control of knowledge and skills

Abbott's (1988) theory of professionalism is concerned with the 'ways occupational groups control knowledge and skill'. The means of gaining control are to emphasize and control techniques and abstract knowledge. This suggests that abstract knowledge has a function other than underpinning practice – it stakes out the territory and marks the power differentials between different occupational groups. For Abbott (1988) the concept of jurisdiction is the central phenomenon of professional life and is the link between the professional and his or her work.

Nursing has since the 1970s been developing its own systematic body of knowledge, so in Freidson's (1970) terms the acquisition of such knowledge would be seen as a professionalization strategy. Larkin (1983), following Freidson, says groups may aspire to professionalism or may think they are professional, 'but they are excluded from a vital component, control of knowledge and its application'. So it is not the gaining of knowledge *per se* that is important, it is how that knowledge is used. Nurse practitioners cannot claim to have their own body of knowledge; their expertise lies in the way knowledge and skills drawn from nursing, medicine, pharmacology, psychology and the physical sciences are brought together in a unique way.

Abbott (1988) suggests that a profession's classification system is a profession's own mapping of its jurisdiction. He takes the system of professions as a structure linking professions with tasks: 'These structural relations bind the professions such that movements of any one affects others.' Thus any movement within medicine can affect nursing. An obvious example of this is the movement to reduce junior doctors' hours, which affects the development of nursing and provided the impetus for the creation of expanded nursing roles in the hospital setting.

Jurisdiction

Abbott uses the term 'jurisdiction' to refer to the rights of a profession to certain modes of action. According to Abbott (1988), there are four components of the professional machinery: diagnosis, inference, treatment and academic knowledge. These elements construct tasks into professional problems, but society has to recognize this by granting the profession claims to exclusive rights. These rights also depend on the social organization of the professions themselves. Abbott (1988, p. 60) contends that:

Claims made in the workplace blur and distort the official lines of legally and publicly established jurisdiction; an important problem for any profession is the reconciliation of its public and workplace position.

Abbott's thesis is concerned with the division of labour; with tasks people see as being in their particular domain and that they claim jurisdiction over. However, these tasks are neither absolute nor permanent, because professions make up an interacting system and therefore the tasks they perform are not static. Furthermore, he argues that 'The subjective qualities of a task arise in the current construction of a problem by the profession currently holding jurisdiction of that task'. So the tasks of assessment, history taking, physical assessment skills, diagnosis, inference and treatment are the core tasks associated with the medical role, and doctors currently hold jurisdiction over diagnosis, inference and treatment, the three acts which Abbott contends are the 'the three acts of professional practice' (regardless of which profession is being discussed).

Diagnosis, according to Abbott, takes information into the professional knowledge system and brings instructions out from it. Inference takes the information of diagnosis and indicates a range of treatments and their predicted outcomes; it is therefore a purely professional act. In this analysis the nurse practitioner can be said to be a true professional because he or she does take the information of diagnosis and from this can conceptualize a range of treatments and their probable outcomes. However, in relation to these core tasks of medicine, the nurse practitioner occupies a contested occupational role within health care. It is a role that is to a large extent controlled by doctors, who ultimately retain the power to decide what is, and what is not, appropriate for nurse practitioners to manage.

The essence of the difference between the nurse practitioner and the doctor therefore, it appears, is in the *degree* to which the nurse practitioner undertakes these professional acts, and this is related to the *complexity* of the presenting conditions dealt with. Linked closely is the amount of *control* the nurse practitioner has regarding work, and the amount of *supervision* he or she is subject to from doctors.

If doctors hold jurisdiction over a task, they can dictate its elements and how it is to be done. If nurses take over a task from doctors, however, they must do so under protocols or clinical guidelines. Once the task has become nurses' work, the subjective qualities of the task become nursing's. Examples of this are wound care, immunizations, cervical cytology, health promotion and screening, all of which are *de facto* part of the nursing role. The aspects of doctors' work that have not yet become routine aspects of nursing work are diagnosis, inference and treatment (including the prescription of medicines); therefore nurses undertake these tasks under controlled conditions and as such can be said to have *discretion* over these domains rather than true autonomy (Witz, 1999, personal communication). This applies also to the prescription of medicines, because only nurses holding a health visiting or district nursing qualification are allowed to prescribe from the *Nurses' Formulary*. However, this is changing as other groups of nurses are now being allowed to prescribe, and at the time of writing the government is seeking guidance from the profession via a consultation exercise completed in January 2001.

It could be argued that rather than having

autonomy, nurse practitioners are allowed a certain amount of discretion in relation to the assessment, diagnosis and management of patients presenting with a narrow range of conditions, and that the discretion that the nurse practitioners have is based on the amount of trust the doctors have in their ability to diagnose and treat correctly, and to know their own limits.

Inference

Identifying signs and symptoms is one thing; knowing what to do about them is another. Just to identify a sign or a symptom, recognize it as a deviation from the norm then refer on does not require in-depth knowledge; it requires a level of practical knowledge sufficient to ensure safe practice. To recognize a sign or symptom as abnormal and then make inferences that lead to treatment requires a deeper level of abstract knowledge and higher-order decision making. Nurse practitioners do more than recognize signs and symptoms and refer straight to a doctor; they also act on their own responsibility in making decisions about management of the problems that patients present with. Many of these problems, it could be argued, do not require a high degree of inference, and that is why doctors allow them to be dealt with by nurse practitioners, for, according to Abbott (1988), too little inference leads to routinization. It is the routine skills of doctors, such as palpation, auscultation and administration of intravenous drugs, that are now often undertaken by nurses, and there is much more routine work that nurses (and others) can undertake instead of doctors. It seems therefore that the subtext is that too much routinization leads to the proletarianization of medical work, which doctors have to resist in order to maintain their exclusive right to power over both patients and para-professionals. However, the defence against wholesale routinization and delegation of diagnosis is that less qualified and experienced workers may miss something serious.

The collecting of evidence on which to base a treatment decision is the diagnosis stage, and Abbott (1988, p. 41) suggests that:

There are rules declaring what kinds of evidence are relevant and irrelevant, valid and invalid, as well as the rules specifying the admissible level of ambiguity.

Abbott says the art of diagnosis is finding the right colligations out of several plausible ones; it is this aspect of diagnosis that doctors claim as their special skill and explains, it seems, why doctors do not like to work to protocols. Protocols place boundaries around diagnosis, inference and treatment, arguably limiting clinical freedom. Furthermore, within the classification system there may be areas of unclassified, residual problems (e.g. tiredness, low mood). These are often labelled as 'trivia' by doctors (Cartwright, 1967) and are seen as appropriate for nurses to deal with, as often what is needed is advice and reassurance rather than specialized treatment. Nurse practitioners taking a leading role with these patients are unlikely to pose a threat to medicine, as they are claiming jurisdiction over an area of medicine that doctors do not value. However, doctors must take care not to be too complacent about their position, as Abbott (1988, p. 47) suggests that: 'Only when a profession has absolute monopoly can it ignore competition.'

Doctors can no longer claim absolute monopoly over diagnosis, inference and treatment. Normally, the more specialized a treatment is, the more the profession is able to maintain jurisdiction over it. An example is chronic disease management, which at one time was treated solely by hospital consultants. Nowadays a range of people manage these conditions, including practice nurses, nurse practitioners, clinical nurse specialists, physio-therapists, occupational therapists and GPs, whilst consultants' jurisdiction is about new treatments and highly specialized therapeutic techniques.

Academic knowledge

Many occupations fight for turf, but only professions expand their dominion by (Abbott, 1988, p. 102):

... using abstract knowledge to annexe new areas – to define them as their own proper work ... abstract knowledge is traditionally central to the claim to professionalism but it is the justification for it that is new. Knowledge is the currency of competition.

In other words, to claim jurisdiction you must first have the appropriate specialized knowledge, but, as was shown earlier, it is not knowledge *per se* that is important, it is knowledge as a resource to be used as a strategy in the quest for professionalization that is important. According to Abbott, academic knowledge is less practical than symbolic, legitimizing professional work by clarifying its foundations and linking them to major cultural values such as service to others. Jurisdiction in the workplace means negotiating around the boundaries of professional jurisdictions, and Abbott (1988, p. 65) argues that jurisdictions tend to disappear in worksites, particularly if those worksites are overworked. This results in the transfer of knowledge, which he calls 'workplace assimilation, in which:

… subordinate professional and members of related equal professions, learn on-the-job a craft version of a given profession's knowledge systems. While they lack the theoretical training that justifies membership in that profession, they generally acquire much of the diagnostic, therapeutic, and inferential systems.

Workplace assimilation, coupled with a theoretically-based course, has helped nurse practitioners to develop the necessary diagnostic, therapeutic and inferential skills required to be effective in their work, but the theoretical base is far less than that of a trained doctor. It is the in-depth knowledge and control over that knowledge that maintain doctor's positions *vis a vis* nurses. However, we need to ask what the function of such knowledge actually is.

Knowledge implies competence, but knowledge quickly becomes out of date and lots of knowledge is forgotten, so knowledge and competence are not the same thing. The boundaries between medical knowledge and nursing knowledge have shifted, the direction of flow being medical knowledge directed towards nurse practitioner, not the other way round. Knowledge can enable and empower incumbents, but the balance must be right; too much is dangerous (for doctors), too little is dangerous (for patients). Turner (1987, p. 135) argues that:

Where the knowledge of the profession is grounded in natural science, this knowledge can become the basis for routine practices. The consequence of this form of knowledge is the fragmentation of the profession and its control by bureaucratic means. It is for this reason that professions need a barrier to protect themselves from such routinization and this barrier is constituted by the indetermination of knowledge; the knowledge of the profession has to have a distinctive mystique which suggests there is a certain professional attitude and competence which cannot be reduced merely to systematic and routinized knowledge. There has to be the development of interpretation which provides the barrier against external regularization through the routinization of its knowledge base.

It is suggested that this barrier can also be used as a form of closure to prevent erosion of medical power by nurse practitioners. Knowledge is used in both an enabling and a constraining way – enabling in that it teaches nurse practitioners what they need to know to accomplish the task, and constraining in that it teaches the limits of their competence but no more than that. It is therefore possible to contend that the nurse practitioner is practising a 'craft version' (Abbott, 1988) of medicine. This is useful to the hospital, as it is an extra skill that can be drawn on when necessary – the nurse practitioner can be used as reserve labour when there is a shortage of doctors. This is an important shift in the division of labour in health care, suggesting that the nurse practitioner is a 'hybrid' health worker (Reveley, 1999).

The transmission of knowledge and how this is done is also relevant. According to Abbott (1988, p. 42), 'dominant professions retain the right to instruct themselves – an important means of domination'. Nursing education, however, was for many years under the influence of medicine. Historically, the education and training of nurses was a contested area within the ranks of nursing itself. On the one hand there were those who perceived nursing as a practical endeavour, and training was to be such as to ensure nurses' competence. Strict discipline, both on the wards and in the nurses' home, would give nurses the confidence to meet the demands of the work. On the other hand, for those fighting for the registration of nurses, training was more than this; it was 'a period of trial to test who was fit to bear the title nurse' (Abel-Smith, 1975).

Training requirements had to be emphasized because of the general belief that every woman could nurse. The longer the period of training and the more demanding it was intellectually, the more the status of nursing would be enhanced. Nursing was to be an elite profession for ladies from a suitable background, and barriers, both financial and educational, should be erected to keep out undesirable recruits. Enhancing the status of nursing by longer and more demanding training would move it along the road of professionalization and thereby gain for nurses some of the privileges enjoyed by doctors, and restricting entry through an exclusionary strategy of closure would create a new subordinate level of lesser skilled workers. The same processes, it can be argued, operate in relation to nurse practitioners, who are carving out some of the 'turf' that previously was within the sphere of competence of medicine, whilst at the same time restricting entry to other nurses by virtue of strict entry criteria and locating the level of nurse practitioner education at Honours or Masters degree level.

The possession of a body of abstract knowledge is also used as a professionalization strategy along with jurisdiction over diagnosis, inference and treatment. It is these elements that are the essence of professional status according to Abbott (1988), and it is these that nurse practitioners are also aspiring to. The question is, how successful are nurse practitioners in achieving 'jurisdiction' (as in Abbott's definition of the term) over these areas of medicine? This question cannot be answered without much more empirical work. However, nurse practitioners have been successful in achieving jurisdiction (or autonomy) over diagnosis, inference and treatment in a great many instances. The context in which nurse practitioners work is vital in this regard. However, as the role is not laid down in statute in the UK, it must be negotiated and reconstituted continuously in every setting where nurse practitioners work. In addition, nurse practitioners require the support of key players in the health care field, and space must be made for them in the internal organization of medicine.

Structural factors that create space for the nurse practitioner role

Abbott (1988) argues that in the system of professions, a profession can seek to dislodge a current incumbent by direct attack, for example by groups entering the system for the first time, or by established groups seeking new turf. Nurse practitioners are the first group of nurses to enter the medical domain to the extent they have, seeking new turf in order to carve out a professional niche for themselves. However, they could not do this if space was not created in the medical domain, and it is factors internal to medicine that have provided this space – such as the internal restructuring of medical work through the junior doctors' hours initiative. Related factors are the increase in chronic conditions heralding the shift from cure to care, the ageing population making increased demands on health care services, increased educational opportunities for nurses, and the increased emphasis on health promotion and prevention. Another factor is external events that serve to eradicate a current jurisdiction, and an example of this is the problem of homeless people who have very limited access to medical care. It was pioneers such as Burke-Masters (1986) who filled the health care gap for this group, and there are now many nurse practitioners working in centres for homeless people. Even this was problematic, however. Burke-Masters came up against severe opposition from medicine and some nurses, which led to her being unable to practise for a year (Burke-Masters, 1988).

Some nurse commentators do not believe that nursing should be about dealing with medicine's internal problems (Keyzer, 1996). On the other hand, if nurses do not undertake those functions that doctors are unable to fill then there is a gap in the service to patients that others will fill to the detriment of nursing.

The social aspect of nursing – creating space for the nurse practitioner?

So how can nurse practitioners claim a professional space that is outside the control of medicine? Davies (1979b) suggests that nurses are often seen as complementing doctors' curative orientation, focusing on more personalized care. The 'new nursing' (Beardshaw and Robinson, 1990) is a means whereby nurses can carve out a separate sphere of competence from medicine. The 'new nursing' came to the fore in the 1970s with the introduction of the nursing process, a concept imported from the USA, which is a problem-solving or 'scientific' approach to nursing care based on assessment, diagnosis, planning, implementation and evaluation of nursing care. It heralded a radical departure from the task-orientated form of nursing practice it replaced, and was not very popular with most doctors and many nurses, being seen as not 'real nursing'. The concept of holism is central to the nursing process, and nurses became concerned with the patient as a whole person, including emotional and social aspects of the patient's life.

The foray into medicine by nurses extending and expanding their roles may be seen as a professionalization strategy, and Salvage (1988) argues that rather than making a bid for traditional professional status, nursing should be seen as a 'new model for occupational authority'.

Salvage (1988, p. 517) believes that:

It is pointless simply to measure the proposals against some arbitrary checklist of professional goals. We should rather assess whether there is a coherent occupational strategy, and if so, which elements of it have persisted and which are responses to rapidly and significantly changed circumstances.

The elements that have persisted are nurses' concern with an holistic patient assessment; concern with the social aspects, health promotion and education; support for clients and carers; and assisting patients to perform those activities of daily living that they would do unaided if able. The elements of the nursing role that are responses to rapidly and significantly changing circumstances are those outlined on the previous page; that is, extended role tasks undertaken under the junior doctors' hours initiative, and the physical assessment skills necessary to provide seamless care to people, particularly those patients who have limited or no access to medical care. As the nurse practitioner role develops, nurse practitioners are dependent on medicine to a large extent for training and support; therefore medicine is in a position of dominance. However, as the role becomes part of primary and hospital-based care, doctors will become dependent on nurse practitioners as they have on other para-professionals (Larkin, 1983). In the meantime, medicine will continue to police the boundary of the nurse practitioner role and boundary maintenance strategies will operate.

Boundary maintenance

When a subordinate group such as nursing becomes essential to work of a superordinate group like doctors, this means that 'maintenance of subordination' occurs (Abbott, 1988); strategies of boundary maintenance are erected. One way to do this is to emphasize the legal boundaries and strengthen the public images of the professions. Thus nurse practitioners' claim to jurisdiction over medical tasks is limited by doctors in the name of medico-legalities. The latter is often illustrated in the popular media, where stereotypes tend to show that all doctors know everything about matters medical and nurses know less than doctors (Abbott, 1988).

Maintenance of subordination also requires the use of symbols such as not wearing a uniform, carrying a stethoscope, having a room of one's own and so on. This poses a dilemma for patients consulting nurse practitioners, as they also have use of these symbols; thus patients have to sort out their interpretation of this situation and staff have to ensure the role of the nurse practitioner is thoroughly publicized (Dowling et al., 1996).

Nurse practitioners have moved quite a way along the road of equality with doctors. However, the structural factors maintaining divisions between medicine and nursing have deep roots, such as the historical development of medicine, which embedded power and status within the profession related to social class and medicine's attachment to 'scientific' knowledge. This is in contrast to the development of nursing, which built on 'craft' knowledge and women's work, and became subordinated to medicine as a by product of nurse reformers' bid for a respectable occupation for women. Furthermore, the patriarchal structures entrenched in Victorian society were reflected in the organization of medicine and nursing and continue to the present, such that gendered strategies of closure (Witz, 1992) continue to operate and power relationships have not altered much over the years.

Conclusion

Nurse practitioners work flexibly, yet also have specialist skills that can be utilized when necessary. As such, they can be said to be carving out a niche for themselves that increases their marketability. However, as we saw in an examination of Abbott's (1988) theory of professionalism, they are taught a craft version of medicine. This, although enhancing their skills and setting them apart from other nurses, limits their autonomy because they do not have full access to the range of medical powers needed for complete autonomy, such as the power to prescribe medication. The work of Abbott (1988) also demonstrated the links between professional autonomy and power, emphasizing the processes at work in establishing and maintaining the powerful position of doctors and the limited power of para-professionals. Medicine and nursing as contested occupational roles are brought into sharp relief by the introduction of the nurse practitioner, as nurse practitioners directly traverse the traditional terrain of doctors and open up a new debate regarding territorial boundaries.

It has been amply demonstrated that nurse practitioners can provide a safe and uncomplicated access route for patients into the health care system, and have both specialist and generalist skills that can be used flexibly. Because of this, nurse practitioners fit well into the changing world of health care, and can be drawn on as reserve army of either nursing or medical labour as the need arises. Nurse practitioners are also at the forefront of the professionalization project of nursing because they have relatively more autonomy and discretion than other nurses; also, because much of the role is negotiated and not bound up in standards of education and practice, it can be creative. This does however raise the question of how the nursing profession deals with the enskilling of qualified nurses and the boundary lines between the enskilling of some and the relatively unchanging role of those at the other end of the scale, who may feel marginalized.

References

Abbott, A. (1988). *The System of Professions: An Essay on the Division of Expert Labour*, pp. 1–102, 315. University of Chicago Press.
Abel-Smith, B. (1975). *A History of the Nursing Profession*, p. 62. Heinemann.
Beardshaw, V. and Robinson, R. (1990). *New for Old? Prospects for Nursing in the 1990s*. King's Fund Institute.
Burke-Masters, B. (1986). The autonomous nurse practitioner: an answer to a chronic problem of primary care. *Lancet*, **1(8492)**, 1266.
Burke-Masters, B. (1988). The nurse in family practice. In: *Nurses and Nurse Practitioners in Primary Health Care* (A. Bowling and B. Stilwell, eds). Scutari Press.
Byrne, P. S. and Long, B. E. (1976). *Doctors Talking to Patients*. HMSO.
Carr-Saunders, A. M. and Wilson, P. (1933). *The Professions*. Clarendon Press.
Cartwright, A. (1967). *Patients and their Doctors*. Routledge and Kegan Paul.
Davies, C. (1979a). Comparative occupational roles in health care. *Social Sci. Med.*, **13a**, 515–21.
Davies, C. (1979b). Organisation theory and the organisation of health care: a comment on the literature. *Social Sci. Med.*, **13a**, 413–22.
Donnison, J. (1977). *Midwives and Medical Men: The Struggle for Control over Childbirth*. Heinemann.
Dowling, S., Martin, R., Skidmore, P. *et al.* (1996). Nurses taking on junior doctors' work: a confusion of accountability. *Br. Med. J.*, **312**, 1211–14.
Durkheim, E. (1964). *The Division of Labour in Society* (trans. G. Simpson). Free Press.
Freidson, E. (1970). *Profession of Medicine*. Dodd Mead.
Gamarnikow, E. (1978). Sexual division of labour: the case of nursing. In: *Feminism and Materialism* (A. Kuhn and A. M. Wolpe, eds), pp. 96–123. Routledge and Kegan Paul.
Hart, N. (1985). The Sociology of Health and Medicine, Ormskirk: Causeway Press.
Johnson, T. (1972). Professions and Power, London: Macmillan.
Keyzer, D. (1996). Keynote speech. Making a World of Difference: Nurse Practitioners, A Global Perspective. Fourth International Conference and Exhibition on Nurse Practitioner Practice, Heriot Watt University, August 22–24.
Larkin, G. V. (1983). *Occupational Monopoly and Modern Medicine*, pp. 1–15. Tavistock.
Larson, M. S. (1977). *The Rise of Professionalism: A Sociological Analysis*. University of California Press.
National Health Service Management Committee (1991). *Junior Doctors: The New Deal*. NHSME.
Parsons, T. (1951). *The Social System*. Free Press.
Reveley, S. (1999). Introducing the nurse

practitioner into general medical practice: theoretical and operational perspectives on the role. Unpublished PhD thesis, University of Lancaster.

Salvage, J. (1988). Professionalisation—or struggle for survival? A consideration of Current Proposals for the Reform of Nursing in the UK. *J. Adv. Nurs.*, **13(4)**, 515–9.

Szasz and Hollender, M. (1956). A Contribution to the Philosophy of Medicine: the Basic Model of the Doctor Nurse Relationship. *Archives on International Medicine*, **97**, 585–92. In: Hart (1985) op. cit.

Turner, B. S. (1987). *Medical Power and Social Knowledge*. Sage.

Weber, M. (1947). The Theory of Social and Economic Organisation, Glencoe: Free Press.

Witz, A, (1992). *Professions and Patriarchy*. Routledge.

Witz, A. (1994). The challenge of nursing. In: *Challenging Medicine* (J. Gabe, D. Kelleher and G. Williams, eds), pp. 23–45. Routledge.

PART 2

Implementing the nurse practitioner role

5

INTRODUCING THE NURSE PRACTITIONER ROLE IN A SURGICAL UNIT: ONE NURSE'S JOURNEY

Shirley Reveley and Kathy Haigh

Introduction

This chapter is about one nurse practitioner's journey from nurse to nurse practitioner. The narrative is a personal one, and what follows is based on an extended, open interview undertaken by the author with the nurse practitioner, and on records kept by the nurse practitioner over a 5-year period from the commencement of her post. It covers the period of her training as a nurse practitioner, and her experiences since qualifying. She practises in a surgical unit located in a district general hospital in the north-west of England. The chapter explores how the role of the nurse practitioner was conceived in this particular hospital unit, and how it developed over time. The aim is to describe the particular experience of one person's transition from nurse to nurse practitioner in order that others may gain insights into developing the nurse practitioner role in the hospital setting. The nurse practitioner's own words are used at certain points in the narrative to illustrate particular issues.

To complete the chapter, a consultant anaesthetist gives his personal view of nurse practitioners and their role.

Surgical nurse practitioner – job description (1995)

1. *Take history (on an agreed protocol basis).*

2. *Pre-admission clinic*:
   - Review patients requiring surgery to assess suitability for anaesthetic and surgical intervention, and identify potential problems (e.g. hypertension, diabetes, chest conditions) that require treatment before surgery is undertaken
   - Liaise with surgeons and anaesthetists to arrange referrals to relevant health professionals to treat problems identified
   - Clerk the patient using a pre-written check-list, and order investigations (ECG, lung function, blood analysis, etc.).

3. *Organize notes and investigations*
   To include barium studies, scan requests, etc. This may involve liaising with the radiologist and X-ray department as required.

4. *Communication*
   With GPs, anaesthetists and other paramedical groups.

5. *Organize discharge summaries and pre-admission discharge planning*
   This includes liaising with nursing staff within the ward environment/clinical area to aid safe discharge of patients into the community or transfers to peripheral hospitals.
   Duties to be undertaken:
   - Completion of discharge summaries
   - Prescription of drugs as per protocol
   - Discharge information for patients
   - Allocation of sick notes
   - Liaison with other paramedical groups as required.

6. *Catheterize patients (male).*

7. *Insert i.v. cannulation.*

8. *Provide a phlebotomy service when phlebotomist is not available.*

9. *Assist in theatre.*

10. *Prescribe drugs and fluids within agreed protocol.*

11. *Assist in outpatient clinics.*

12. *Assist junior doctors with their duties.*

13. *Educate patients and staff in general surgery developments and health promotion.*

14. *Participate in clinical audit.*

15. *Initiate and participate in any research proposal.*

Title

The nurse practitioner described here uses the title 'nurse practitioner: general surgery'. She was one of the first nurse practitioners to be employed by the hospital Trust, and commenced the post in November 1995. Nobody at the time in the surgical unit knew what nurse practitioners really were or what they did. The nurse practitioner herself was unsure of exactly what the role entailed. Another nurse practitioner had been appointed in neurology a month previously; however, the neurological and the surgical nurse practitioner roles developed very differently.

The first job description (1995)

The role of the 'nurse practitioner: general surgery' was created in response to the reduction in junior doctors' hours initiative (NHSME, 1991; Loveland, 1992; Read and Graves, 1994). It was envisaged that the nurse practitioner would reduce the junior doctors' workload and ultimately help with decreasing their hours. What was wanted initially was a nurse specialist to work on the wards, undertaking an extended role including procedures such as cannulation of patients and taking arterial blood gases. The job description (see box on page 51) included history taking, against an agreed protocol, in order that the nurse practitioner would be able to undertake the junior doctors' role on the ward. This reflected a task-orientated approach, but was not what the nurse practitioner herself believed the role should be, as it was too medicalized. Nurse practitioner as doctor substitute roles are described in the literature but are not well supported (Ford and Walsh, 1994); they do little for advancing nursing practice and demean the nurses' knowledge and skills (Castledine, 1994). However, once in post the nurse practitioner was advised that the job description was only a template from which she could practise initially. The development of the role was placed firmly in her hands; how she advanced the role was for her to investigate, and any change would be based on patient need and the needs of the organization. The nurse practitioner wished to see an expansion of the nursing role; she did not want to become a technical functionary or lose her expert clinical skills. It could be argued that technical aspects of care are as relevant as nursing functions, and together they provide a true holistic approach to the patient. However, to provide the technical aspects of care outside a nursing framework fragments patient care. Unqualified healthcare assistants can be trained to provide a phlebotomy or cannulation service, but such roles represent a task-orientated approach and do not allow for the intervention that is nursing.

Reactions from colleagues

The major difficulty in the early days was related to poor definition of the role; no one understood what a nurse practitioner was, or how a nurse practitioner functioned. The UKCC in the final report on PREP (UKCC, 1994) did not recognize the term nurse practitioner, and still does not. The probable reasons for this are discussed elsewhere (Reveley, 1999). Furthermore, great debate surrounds the concept of levels of nursing practice; what constitute 'specialist' or 'advanced' nursing roles? Can these be concepts be adequately captured? For a fuller discussion, see Woods (2000).

Some medical staff were wary of this nurse, who was initially perceived as 'doing a doctor's job', and they could see no need for such a person. Some nursing colleagues were very sceptical of the role, and their comments were at times derogatory in nature. Hupcey (1993) found that one of the main barriers working against nurse practitioner development was the attitude of professional colleagues, particularly staff nurses. The nurse practitioner herself sought to understand the concept of the nurse practitioner through the literature, using Stilwell et al.'s (1987) characteristics of a nurse practitioner, which are:

- Accountability for professional practice
- Autonomous practice
- Clinical decision making
- Instigating treatment based on decisions
- Patient advocacy
- Teamworking.

She disseminated this information to her colleagues, who were not always convinced – as the following incident demonstrates:

> A nurse berated me for leaving nursing and trying to be a 'mini doctor', she stated that I should 'have the guts to go to medical school and do it properly'. This had been instilled in the staff of the ward and they were very unreceptive to the change. Their minds had been set and what faced me was a long haul to change their opinions and 'prove' that nursing was still the driving force and philosophy behind this new, exciting role.—*Nurse Practitioner*

The argument as to whether nurse practitioners are merely doctor substitutes has been ongoing for a long time, and antagonists of the role would support the contention (Emmerson, 1996), whilst others vigorously refute it (Cable, 1994; Emmerson, 1996). The nurse practitioner discussed in this chapter sees her work as combining medical and nursing roles; she insists that her work is not that of doctor substitute. In her own words:

> I had the confidence to go for it because that's what I knew I wanted to do and knew where I wanted to go. It was new, it was exciting and I thought 'Oh, yes, I fancy that', and because of the background that I'd had, that I'd worked autonomously for a long time, albeit with a group of nurses, we worked autonomously within that group, I felt that I really could bring medicine and nursing together. I never at any stage felt that I was taking on a doctor's role. My thoughts have always been that I am a nurse, first and foremost, and all I've done is bring a bit of medicine into nursing. I have not taken nursing into medicine. If I had wanted to be a doctor, I would have gone to medical school.—*Nurse Practitioner*

She sees herself then as bringing medicine into nursing and bringing nursing and medicine together. This combining of roles constitutes a new, hybrid health worker (Reveley, 1999).

Initially the nurse practitioner did not feel supported in her new role by some of her colleagues, and reported that at times she felt she was in a lonely position. However, support was evident from some clinical nurse specialists in the hospital. They described to her their experiences of introducing a new role, the barriers they had met and how these were overcome:

The clinical nurse specialists that were already in post were extremely supportive. They said: 'you'll not know what you're doing for at least 6 months, but don't worry about it. Take everybody with a pinch of salt because they won't know what they want you to do either'. They helped and guided us and they were very helpful. There were times when they couldn't help because they didn't understand where we were supposed to be going either because there wasn't a great deal written down.

Relationships with other health professionals

There were issues regarding the referral of patients to other agencies within the multidisciplinary team. Traditionally nursing staff had assessed the need for intervention by other agencies, but requests for such interventions had to be signed for by a doctor. This seemed a ludicrous situation, and one the nurse practitioner intended to rectify. Following discussions with the relevant departments, they agreed to nurse practitioner referrals, provided that the nurse practitioner took responsibility for such requests. This enabled requests to be made much faster. The ability to refer to other health care professionals improved the service for the patients. For example, those patients who were to undergo major surgery could be seen pre-operatively and given a high protein diet for a few days prior to admission. Those with pulmonary problems could have their condition optimized by attending for pre-operative chest physiotherapy for a week. It opened the floodgates of opportunity for ensuring that the patients were well prepared both physically and emotionally for their impending surgery.

Ordering X-rays

It was acknowledged that as part of an holistic assessment of the patient the nurse may have to request a chest X-ray, but this proposal to the radiology directorate was met with much opposition. Rules and regulations regarding who could request X-rays and who could not were cited, and it was argued that nurses fell into the group who could not. Eventually the radiologists stated they would support the nurse practitioner if she undertook the Radiation Protection Course and requested

X-rays following the guidelines laid down by the Society of Radiographers. She did undertake the required course and developed the knowledge necessary to request X-rays; however, she has to identify on the request card that it is a nurse practitioner request. This service has been audited and it has been found that she requests fewer X-rays than most junior doctors, and of those that are requested 60 per cent have an abnormality when reported on. It is interesting to note here that the hospital employs emergency nurse practitioners who have not been allowed to request X-rays. The knowledge that one nurse in a different department had been granted permission caused a period of consternation and turmoil for the nurse practitioner:

> We were the first two nurses in the north west who were given permission to request X-rays of chest and abdomen. In this hospital the A&E nurse practitioner still can't request X-rays. We asked, 'why can't we do it?' and were told, 'because you're nurses'. We said 'Well, what do we need to know to be able to do it?' and were advised to go on the Radiation Protection Course. So we went and did it, at a regional teaching hospital; we came back and said, 'we've done it, can we order X-rays now?'. It's called the Radiation Protection Course for Nurses, and I do suggest that any nurse who wants to request X-rays goes on it, because I don't think you quite realize what goes on, not just the requesting X-rays; it's how much radiation is given to the patient and whether an X-ray is really necessary.—*Nurse Practitioner*

Preparation for the role: starting again

Patricia Benner (1984) describes how nurses pass through a series of stages that begin at novice level, and continue through proficiency to arrive at expert levels of nursing practice. This particular nurse practitioner had 10 years' experience working with surgical patients before taking up her new post, and therefore believed herself to be practising at an expert level in her sphere. However, when faced with a new role she felt that she had 'lost' her knowledge and became a novice once more. Benner (1984) states that any nurse who changes an area of practice returns to the

novice state for a period of time, whilst he or she consolidates experience and transfers this to the new sphere of practice. This feeling stayed with the nurse practitioner for several months whilst she consolidated her knowledge and learnt new skills.

There is little in the published literature on the experience of nurse practitioners as they make the transition from nursing into this advanced role. However, one study (Brown and Olshansky, 1997) describes the experiences of 35 nurse practitioners in the first year following completion of their nurse practitioner programme in the USA. They were interviewed three times over the year, and analysis of the interviews revealed 'a process of professional development that unfolded during the first year following graduation'. The authors say this process is reflected in the theoretical model 'from limbo to legitimacy' (Brown and Olshansky, 1997). There is a slow emergence over time from identity confusion – straddling two identities and not feeling part of either – to taking on the identity of nurse practitioner. These new nurse practitioners experienced many obstacles to establishing their new identity, but 1 year post-qualifying, although still learning and developing, they had gained enough experience to be comfortable in their new role and see themselves as legitimate nurse practitioners.

Skill development

The nurse practitioner was a very experienced nurse who had previously worked in a renal unit, where she had undertaken a relatively autonomous role. For the first 6 months of her new post she worked with a surgical consultant, helping to look after the patients – for example, helping to update discharge letters, making sure that all the information was going where it ought to, and improving the standard of the discharge letter. She then began giving the patients more information, both pre-operatively and post-operatively, whilst learning how to examine patients physically, working to protocols and working alongside the doctors, with the consultants. As more experience was gained in physical examination, her confidence developed and the nurse practitioner began to recognize deviations from the norm, although diagnosis at this stage was not attempted. A systems approach was taken to learning, and each body system was learnt thoroughly, together with correct techniques for examining that system. If a problem was discovered, the patient was immediately passed on to a doctor.

Thus the nurse practitioner underwent a period of in-house training to equip her with the skills and knowledge to fulfil the role. In order to facilitate skills development, the hospital nominated a medical facilitator to teach physical examination skills in relation to surgical patients. Although grateful for this opportunity, the nurse practitioner felt it was not sufficient to ensure that she was a safe and competent practitioner; there was a need for some educational underpinning in order to demonstrate credibility. There was also a need for a more structured and consistent approach to history taking and physical examination of patients. Furthermore, there was little theory underpinning the practical skills, and on reflection, if she had continued with this type of training, the nurse practitioner felt she would not be adhering to the UKCC's *Scope of Professional Practice* (UKCC, 1992a) or the *Code of Professional Conduct* (UKCC, 1992b). The legal aspect of nursing has been well-described by Dimond (1990), who states that as well as a professional responsibility to the UKCC, the nurse is also accountable in both civil and criminal law. Ford and Walsh (1994) point out that this has implications for education and training in the nurse practitioner role. They describe education as:

Developing a flexible enquiring mind able to approach a situation from different angles. The individual should be able to consider alternative solutions within a critical and analytical framework, utilizing a strong knowledge base, before deciding on a solution to a problem or a course of action.

The nurse practitioner voiced her concerns about her training and investigated the availability of educational courses for nurse practitioners. Subsequently she embarked on the BSc (Hons) Nurse Practitioner day-release programme, to equip her with the educational theory and practical skills that would underpin her practice and allow her to develop into a safe, competent and holistic nurse practitioner. The design and content of the nurse practitioner degree programme provided the nurse practitioner with knowledge that was firmly rooted in nursing philosophy. It encouraged her to seek different ways of approaching patient care whilst remaining a safe and competent practitioner, and at the same time teaching skills of assessment. This education, along with additional clinical support from the medical facilitator, allowed the nurse to become competent in some aspects of physical examinations. Throughout the course of her work the nurse practitioner was assessed by her facilitator (on her request) to assess the levels of competencies attained. Following successful completion of assessments, she felt able to instigate nurse-led clinics. The nurse practitioner was aware of her level of competence and followed protocols (written at local level) which acted as risk assessment tools. These protocols addressed patients' suitability for anaesthesia and allowed the nurse practitioner to assess the patient and refer on when necessary for medical management.

Barriers to implementing the role

The attitude of some health professionals towards the role are highlighted above, but the nurse practitioner in the interview revealed that a big barrier to be overcome was an initial a loss of confidence in her own ability. The following extract from the interview illustrates this well:

When I first started this job I felt that because of my years in surgery, not only did I work in the renal unit, but I had a part-time job on the surgical unit anyway and always have had my hand in with surgery, I felt from an ego point of view, an expert – a clinical/surgical nurse. The day I took my uniform off and put on my own clothes to become a nurse practitioner, I lost that and I felt naked, stripped, pathetic, like I didn't have any knowledge whatsoever and everything had gone and I was this little person, stood there thinking I don't know anything, I know nothing. It took me 3 months to actually realize that I still knew how to nurse patients, but I was going through one of those gigantic learning curves where I was a novice nurse practitioner, but an expert nurse. It was very, very difficult. That was when I really did have a crisis of confidence. I hadn't read Benner's work then. I read that book from cover to cover and the identification made me wish I'd read it earlier, because it made me feel ... that I was an expert at one thing, a novice at another and then having to rebuild my confidence.—*Nurse Practitioner*

Arena and Page (1992) state that clinical nurse specialists in the acute care setting may feel unprepared for their role as 'all round experts'. They may become depressed, lose self-confidence and feel uneducated. These and other feelings, they argue, may lead to an experience of the 'imposter phenomenon'. This is a term that has been used to describe those individuals who achieve success but have hidden feelings of inadequacy regarding their achievements. They do not accept that they are intelligent, and feel they are fooling people. There is a particularly high incidence of this phenomenon in women achievers. It is thought that the root of these feelings may lie in social expectations of women wherein women are not defined as competent (Clance and Imes, 1978). This is an interesting line of discussion, and the feelings described by Arena and Page are not dissimilar to those reported by nurse practitioner students.

However, with increased knowledge and skills the nurse practitioner regained confidence and, as she became more secure in her role, started a pre-admission clinic. As the following extract shows, she still required a lot of support:

When I started the nurse practitioner-led pre-admission clinic, I was just becoming a confident practitioner, not an expert, I was in no way the person I am today. I was a novice nurse practitioner, requiring a lot of support from the doctors. I needed somebody on the end of the phone, just in case. Sometimes to validate what I'd found, because I wasn't sure. The balance I would have said was 70 per cent in favour of getting somebody else to check, 30 per cent my own clinical judgement and trust in myself. The balance has swung the other way now, probably 30 per cent of the time I would ring someone and 70 per cent of the time it's my own clinical skills and judgement, and I stand by my decisions and have a rationale behind the decisions I make.—*Nurse Practitioner*

Responding to need

The literature on nurse practitioner development points to the role being introduced in response to an identified gap in services, often the lack of appropriate medical care in a particular location, or for a particular client group (Burke-Masters, 1986; Fawcett-Henesy, 1991). Once in post, nurse practitioners find opportunities to develop and shape the role further, often in response to the needs of their patients. This nurse practitioner was no different:

A need was identified within the surgical unit to set up a nurse-led pre-admission clinic for patients in order to reduce the amount of inappropriate admissions, facilitate the appropriate use of resources, and to provide an enhanced service to the patients. Pre-admission clinics are not a new concept. Though the nurse practitioner felt able to carry out nursing and social assessment of patients, she believed it to be inappropriate to set up such a clinic with her limited knowledge and felt unable to carry out physical examinations for which she had very little knowledge and skills. The nurse practitioner therefore read widely to increase her knowledge in both the medical and nursing care of concurrent medical problems that a patient may present with, such as diabetes, asthma, hypertension and coronary heart disease. This allowed her to assess patients' fitness for anaesthesia and give advice and health education. It also increased her self-confidence. Importantly, she had access to a consultant at all times and recognized the limits of her knowledge and sought advice whenever needed.

Once the pre-admission clinics were implemented a whole range of opportunities opened up for the nurse practitioner. Not only is there time for health assessment, but there is also time for educating the patients and increasing awareness of health education issues. Patients who are anxious have time to voice their fears and concerns. On occasions, patients have talked of other issues and counselling has followed. The value of pre-admission clinics may be measured in terms of cost savings to the organization for inappropriate admissions. However, it is difficult to measure the additional services of counselling apart from patient satisfaction surveys.

This service, in the nurse practitioner's view, does not present a 'medicalized' role; rather, it presents an opportunity for a holistic approach to service delivery by providing both a nursing and a medical function. This enhances the nurse–patient relationship and is firmly rooted in nursing philosophy.

In terms of the degree course, the nurse practitioner underwent a huge learning curve. Modules were relevant to advanced nursing practice and allowed the nurse practitioner to explore new methods of patient care. The course enabled her to become more analytical and explore new ways of approaching problems. A lasting memory of the first year of the course is the peer support provided by the fellow students; it was comforting to be aware that all were undergoing a period of change and uncertainty. The course provided excellent role models, in that it was mainly taught by qualified nurse practitioners, some with years of experience, who facilitated

---

Main duties and responsibilities of the nurse practitioner – job description (1997)

1. Participate and manage a defined caseload of nurse-led clinics, including pre-admission clinics and anaesthetic assessments:
   - Take history and perform physical examination, take blood samples, make requests for ECGs, bloods, X-rays, etc., and provide pre- and post-operative information, counselling, health education and advice
   - Take responsibility for decisions made regarding patient care
   - Liaise with surgeons, anaesthetists and nursing staff
   - Liaise with medical secretaries and waiting list manager
   - Provide excellent documentation and ensure all relevant information is included.

2. Provide inpatient services, including:
   - Cannulation and venepuncture
   - Arterial blood sampling
   - Male catheterization
   - ECG recording
   - Insertion of fine-bore nasogastric tubes
   - Prescription of items defined by Crown protocols
   - Provision of discharge information to general practitioners
   - Discharge of patients from the service.

3. Provide counselling (where no other specialist nursing services exist), health education and advice to patients, relatives and carers.

4. Provide and manage a telephone help line service for patients and carers.

5. Provide and manage post-operative wound care clinics, including:
   - Accepting referrals from nurses and consultants
   - Carrying own caseload of patients
   - Taking responsibility for patients' care
   - Making autonomous decisions re wound management
   - Liaising with tissue viability nurse as appropriate
   - Discharging patients from the service
   - Communicating with GPs and district nurses.

6. Participate in the expansion of nurse-led clinics and services and manage workload as appropriate.

7. Ensure appropriate referrals are made to both internal and external agencies as required.

8. Develop close working relationships with surgeons, anaesthetists and ward staff to ensure good continuity of care for patients.

9. Provide evidence-based education and training to all staff to enhance standards of care.

10. Act as a resource for colleagues and outside agencies.

11. Research, develop and implement evidence-based guidelines for both nursing and medical staff.

12. Participate in and initiate research projects; evaluate and report findings.

13. Implement and manage change to improve standards of care.

14. Continuously develop your own knowledge and skills, with an emphasis on evidence-based practice.

15. Prioritize work to meet both personal and organizational objectives.

16. Undertake audits of nurse practitioner activities and produce reports.

17. Undertake annual patient satisfaction surveys, produce reports and action plans to improve services.

the transition from nurse to student nurse practitioner. The first year made the student nurse practitioner more aware of the issues surrounding the role. It gave her the knowledge required to convince her colleagues, both nursing and medical, to accept that the role was here to stay, and that it was having a beneficial effect on both the patients and the organization.

The second job description (1997)

This was written in the second year of practice and was in stark contrast to the first job description (see box on page 57). Although the medical tasks remained, 'assist junior doctors with their duties' was removed and replaced with 'act as a resource for colleagues and outside agencies' to enable them to provide a continuity of care consistent with current guidelines. As the pre-admission service gained recognition, so did the role of the nurse practitioner. No longer was the role viewed as task-orientated; it was accepted as an holistic approach to patient care. Subsequently the job description changed to incorporate all the aspects of the role, followed by re-grading and monetary reward in recognition of the efforts of the nurse practitioner. The role became more autonomous, with additions to the nurse practitioner's sphere of practice.

With the co-operation of consultants, a post-operative wound care clinic was started. This was to reduce clinic visits by patients who had chronic unhealed wounds. The nurse practitioner assessed, implemented and evaluated patients' care, and discharged them from the service. Soon after its inception, consultants were readily referring patients to this clinic and were calling on the nurse practitioner for advice regarding wound care for patients on the ward. This led to consultants referring on some of their domiciliary visits to patients who required surgical debridement of wounds. The nurse practitioner then had the additional responsibility of assessing these patients and arranging admission if she thought it necessary. Autonomous decisions were thus being taken by the nurse practitioner, with she having sole responsibility for the care of this group of patients. The service was audited to ensure that she was making the correct

decisions, and the audit demonstrated that this was so in 96 per cent of cases admitted for surgical debridement. Of those that she did not admit, she had made the correct decision in 97 per cent of cases. The nurse practitioner felt encouraged by these results because it demonstrated that she was sufficiently competent. The consultants and the organization agreed with this.

This success represented a leap in the professional development of the nurse practitioner, who now felt she had advanced along the path described by Benner (1984) to becoming a proficient nurse practitioner who was striving to attain expert clinical practice. Ford and Walsh (1994) state that the key to excellence is:

Allowing the nurse to develop and grow individually, building their expertise on feedback from experience, rather than procedure manuals. The nurse is free to take reasonable risks and allowed from time to time to fail. Failure is then used as a positive learning experience as the nurse reflects on why things did not work out.

Ford and Walsh (1994) describe this as a positive feedback loop, as practice then feeds reflection in action, innovation and creativity, which in turn leads to expert care. However, the role was still not without problems because, for example, the community nurses were concerned that a nurse was 'doing a doctor's job'. Once the role of the nurse practitioner, how this role enhanced patient care, and that she was not there to threaten them in any way, had been explained, they became more co-operative. The nurse practitioner expanded the service to include domiciliary visits for patients who were disabled and found it difficult to return to clinic for wound care.

The educational input in the second year was a valuable asset to the nurse practitioner's knowledge base, particularly the pharmacology module, which gave her further insight into the use of medication and its actions. It allowed her to speak to patients with greater knowledge on how the drugs they were taking worked, and to cascade the information learned by her to colleagues. She took on an educative role in the Intravenous Drug Administration study days run by the surgical unit. This demonstrates the professional growth of the nurse practitioner, as does the example of how competence and confidence was developed:

> The nurse practitioner wanted to follow up patients post-discharge. This would ensure that in some cases the nurse practitioner would have seen them pre-operatively, during their stay in hospital, and again post-operatively. This would enhance continuity of care for the patients and reduce the amounts of patients seen in clinic by the consultant. In order to prepare herself for this additional sphere of practice, the nurse practitioner spent 6 months 'shadowing' a registrar in the outpatient clinic and, under supervision, made decisions regarding management or discharge of these patients. This was a period of intense learning, and at times the nurse practitioner felt insecure in her knowledge and acknowledged that she needed more time to feel truly confident in her actions. This resonates with the UKCC's *Code of Professional Conduct* document, which states that the nurse must ensure that her actions do not have any detrimental effect on the patient and that the nurse should recognize her limitations and decline responsibility until she feels competent and confident in her decisions. Thus the nurse practitioner continued to work under supervision for another period of 6 months in order to enhance her knowledge and skills.

During the third year of her post, further opportunities presented themselves for the nurse practitioner. There had been a period of knowledge consolidation, and the nurse practitioner was able to move away from the restrictive protocols that had guided her through the first and second years of practice. Benner (1984) describes how experienced nurses are able to look beyond the presenting problem and use problem-solving approaches different from those of a novice nurse. The experienced nurse is able to consolidate prior experiences as a whole and apply them to different situations without wasteful considerations of irrelevant material (Dreyfus and Dreyfus, 1980). The nurse practitioner's knowledge and expertise were evident in this stage of development, and she was aware that she was tackling problems both analytically and intuitively. She was able to 'see' problems that patients did not perceive as problems. This is what Benner (1984) describes as 'intuitive' nursing. For example, a patient's body language may not be consistent with the spoken responses, suggesting an underlying problem. A nurse intuitively knows when something is not quite right, but is sometimes unable to vocalize exactly what is wrong.

Developing autonomy

As mentioned above, the nurse practitioner moved away from the restrictive protocols that had been previously written. It was acknowledged by the organization that she had developed skills in advance of their expectations, and she was therefore encouraged to develop her role further. The restrictive protocols were removed and in their place were guidelines for practice, which gave greater scope for practice. For example, initially if a patient had been found to be unsuitable for anaesthesia, the nurse practitioner had to refer the patient to the consultant for review before the patient was taken off the list for surgery. The new guidelines encouraged the nurse practitioner to use her own clinical judgement to make the decision to remove a patient from the list. It also allowed for her to explore different treatment options with the patient. For example:

> A patient with a large inguinal hernia with co-existing airways disease who was on constant oxygen was not suitable for any operative intervention. He agreed that operation was not an option, but different treatment options were discussed, with the patient being left to make the final decision. The non-medical option was a truss. The patient agreed to try this option and, on review, the patient stated that he had no symptoms from his hernia.

This example demonstrates how the nurse practitioner has not just taken on a medical role, but has also enhanced her nursing role to include medicine and is therefore able to offer alternative forms of treatment which enhance patient comfort.

The role finally achieved recognition within the surgical unit, and attitudes towards the role of the nurse practitioner have changed. There is a general acceptance that pre-admission clinics have enhanced patient services and decreased the amount of inappropriate admissions, and have also achieved a higher standard of pre-operative discharge planning, which reduces the length of stay for patients. Patients are reported to be less anxious and more knowledgeable on admission to hospital, and more aware of length of stay, expectations of treatment and post-operative restrictions. Thus patients are empowered within the health care system. Clay (1991) describes empowerment as 'helping clients and patients to take control of their own destiny and understand their own health needs'. By giving patients information regarding their operations, they are better prepared for their surgery and their recovery.

The educational input continued and equipped the nurse practitioner with more than just the technical skill of physical examination; it taught her to be reflective, inquisitive and constructively critical, which Ford and Walsh (1994) state is as important as developing communication and interpersonal skills, research, innovative management and leadership skills. They also fear that if the education is fixed on the medical model, the nurse practitioner initiative will have failed. Demonstration of competence is a key feature of acceptance of the nurse practitioner role and, as stated by the nurse practitioner herself, this is clearly the case in this particular instance:

> Once the practical examinations had been completed there was a change in the attitudes of the medical staff. Credibility in their eyes had been achieved. They acknowledged the achievement of the nurse practitioner and one consultant in particular stated that he did not know how the service had managed in the past without a nurse practitioner. This was a complete change from the initial statement made by the same consultant earlier in the development of the role.—*Nurse Practitioner*

Measuring success

Success means different things to different people, and thus there are multiple perspectives on success depending upon whose point of view is sought. A variety of interests are represented when introducing a new nursing role (Smith and Cantley, 1985), such as the interests of patients, managers, doctors, therapists, nurses and the relatives of patients. A formal evaluation project needs to take account of these interests. However, there was no formal evaluation of the introduction of the nurse practitioner role in this particular organization. Nevertheless, success can be assessed through less formal means, and the nurse practitioner soon realized that, although a novice at this role, she could make a significant difference to the delivery of a service for the patients. It soon became evident that the service was successful in terms of the decrease in the number of operations cancelled, and the fact that patients were vocal in their support for this new initiative. The professional group most affected by this change was the anaesthetists, who supported the service from its inception. They reported a significant decrease in the number of patients being declined anaesthesia due to inadequate pre-operative preparation.

In a general survey of patients who have attended pre-admission clinics, all stated they would have no objections to seeing the nurse practitioner post-operatively. Other recent initiatives implemented by the nurse practitioner include reducing the number of telephone calls made to wards in the early post-operative period. She has set up a telephone help-line for patients with queries following operation. Each patient has the telephone number of the help-line printed on the bottom of the discharge information sheet provided. Following the implementation of this initiative, the ward staff have reported a decrease in the amount of telephone calls received. The nurse practitioner has had many calls from patients, all of which required some nursing information, or general information to be given. Again this has increased patient satisfaction, because patients know to whom they are talking and can relate to the nurse practitioner, who they have met previously. The role of nurse practitioner has now been accepted throughout the hospital and is having a direct impact on patient care. Patient need has always been the driving force behind the development of the role. It is of interest here to demonstrate how the service has been accepted and is now commonplace.

Whilst the nurse practitioner was on annual leave for 2 weeks, there were seven cancelled operations due to inadequate preparation for anaesthetic (there is no cover for pre-admission clinics whilst the nurse practitioner is away). The nurse practitioner felt an acute sense of responsibility for this breakdown of service. She has for some time tried to demonstrate the need for a further nurse practitioner and now has the evidence to 'prove' that nurse practitioners do indeed make a significant contribution to patient care. She now has responsibility for waiting list initiatives for minor surgery, e.g. hernias and varicose veins. She assesses suitability for anaesthesia, discusses with patients when they would like the operation to be carried out and places patients on theatre lists, all without involvement of a doctor. This is truly a nurse-led service. Of course, the nurse practitioner communicates with the appropriate surgeon and anaesthetist regarding these patients, and there is an acceptance by them that the patients will have been well prepared and do not need any further intervention by themselves.

The future

The nurse practitioner now wants to provide continuity of care by reviewing patients post-operatively. This is soon to become reality for,

---

Nurse practitioner in general surgery (for newly appointed nurse practitioners) – job description (2000)

Job purpose:
To work closely with the established nurse practitioner in general surgery. This is an additional post to support the increasing surgical services workload. The primary function is to provide specialist nursing services to general surgical patients, both pre- and post-operatively.

Main duties and responsibilities:
1. Maintain the nurse practitioner service in general surgery:
   - In collaboration with other nurse practitioners in general surgery, participate in a defined caseload of nurse-led pre-assessment clinics and anaesthetic assessments
   - Provide post-operative wound care clinics, liaising with nurses, consultants, patients, GPs and district nurses
   - Provide a telephone help-line service to patients and carers
   - Provide specialist inpatient clinical services as required – e.g. cannulation and venepuncture, arterial blood sampling, male catheterization, ECG recording, insertion of fine-bore nasogastric tubes.
2. Maintain a healthy, safe and productive working environment following legislative and clinical requirements.
3. Contribute to the environment of the nurse practitioner services in general surgery:
   - Review the services provided and implement changes required to continuously improve patient care
   - Participate in the expansion of the nurse-led clinics and other specialist services.
4. Optimize the use of resources to provide an effective service to patients:
   - Make recommendations for the use of resources, including time, room availability, bed usage, equipment and consumables
   - Plan the use of physical resources, in particular clinic services and facilities
   - Obtain the necessary resources to provide a general standard of patient care.
5. Enhance your own performance by maintaining your licence to practise:
   - Continuously develop your knowledge and skills by attending conferences and professional meetings, and by reading professional journals and published research
   - Participate in and initiate research projects and evidence-based practice; evaluate report findings
   - Optimize your own resources in relation to self-management, delegating and prioritizing work.
6. Gain the trust and support of colleagues, including surgeons, anaesthetists, ward staff and medical secretaries.
7. Contribute to the learning and development of colleagues and outside agencies to enhance standards of care for patients.
8. Provide accurate and complete information to facilitate patient care, including referrals to internal and external agencies and the discharge of patients:
   - Educate and train staff in new service developments and clinical practices to improve patient care to surgical patients
   - Provide health education and advice to patients, relatives and carers
   - Provide written and verbal reports on research findings, audit reports and patient satisfaction surveys.

with further education and guidance, she now feels confident in the management of these patients. Guidelines are being prepared for the implementation of this much-needed service. From an organizational viewpoint this service could not be implemented at a better time because there has been a steep increase in the number of new patient referrals – so much so that one consultant has had to increase the number of clinic sessions available. Through providing this service the nurse practitioner will contribute to the reduction in waiting times for new patients to be seen by the surgical team. More nurse practitioners are now being employed in general surgery in this hospital to help meet demand.

The third job description (2000)

See box on page 61.

Advice to others wanting to become nurse practitioners

The nurse practitioner featured here gives the following advice to those wanting to undertake the role:

1. Be confident in what you're doing, but don't try to run before you can walk.
2. Inform and educate colleagues and clients about the role.
3. Remember that whatever you do you are accountable for your actions, so make sure that what you do enhances patient care.
4. Make sure that you audit the service.
5. Evaluate the service you offer from the patient's point of view.
6. Explain what a nurse practitioner is, because patients don't know. Wear a badge. All letters sent out to patients should state that they will be seeing a nurse practitioner.
7. Give patients the choice of seeing the nurse practitioner or the doctor.
8. Keep careful records.

Conclusion

This chapter has given an account of one nurse practitioner's journey from nurse to nurse practitioner. It has been a challenging but ultimately rewarding process. Changing attitudes and beliefs towards the role has been difficult, but the role has now been accepted as an integral part of the nursing/medical team. This nurse practitioner's story is one that is being repeated all over the country in different locations and in numerous clinical settings. For nurse practitioners to be successful and gain the respect of peers, patients and managers, they have to be persistent, dedicated, knowledgeable and skilled. This particular nurse practitioner has demonstrated all these characteristics and shown that introducing a nurse practitioner service into the acute setting does indeed enhance the service to patients and clients.

Finally, there follows a personal view of the nurse practitioner by a consultant anaesthetist.

The surgical nurse practitioner – a personal view from a consultant anaesthetist

[The following commentary is provided by Nick Harper, Consultant Anaesthetist, Blackpool Victoria NHS Trust]

My personal experience of working with nurse practitioners is in the field of pre-anaesthetic and pre-operative assessment. Whilst I am fully aware that my nurse practitioner colleagues interface in many other areas – wound care, for example – my involvement in those areas is minimal.

Anaesthetic pre-assessment has invariably been a rather grey area. Whilst the anaesthetist performs a pre-operative visit and a formal anaesthetic assessment, this is often on the same day as the operation. Clearly any significant problem encountered at this stage will frequently lead to surgery being delayed or postponed. In order to detect problems earlier many surgeons perform a pre-assessment themselves, in the surgical outpatient clinic, and then contact the anaesthetist should advice be needed. Unfortunately this type of assessment is often brief and hurried, and it is not surprising that medical and anaesthetic conditions are missed under these circumstances. Thus problems still come to light on the day of surgery despite the best efforts of the surgeons.

Nurse practitioners performing anaesthetic

pre-assessment and surgical pre-operative assessment have a dedicated role. It is their responsibility to ensure that patients are as well as they can be. This role includes some assessment of chronic conditions, and also screening for medical problems, relevant but not yet detected. Such problems could cause cancellation on the day of surgery due to the need of further investigation and/or treatment pre-operatively.

The benefit of this service to the surgeon is a reduction in operation cancellations on the day of surgery. Furthermore, patients pre-assessed by the nurse practitioner do not require lengthy formal clerking by the surgical house officer, thus freeing them to perform other duties. The benefit for the anaesthetist is a patient who has been assessed reliably and to a consistent standard, who will be appropriately worked up for theatre and well informed.

As an anaesthetist I find nurse practitioners to be highly motivated, talented, interested and helpful members of the peri-operative team. They detect problems and arrange investigations appropriately, within given guidelines and protocols. When necessary they will then contact the anaesthetist to discuss the patient, surgery and anaesthetic (with all the relevant information and results on hand). On occasion they contact the anaesthetist for advice on how to proceed with a given patient. It may be essential that the anaesthetist perform a formal pre-operative anaesthetic assessment, and nurse practitioners are key in identifying such patients.

So far I have described the role of nurse practitioner as that of a well-motivated and well-trained surgical house officer! It is true that the roles overlap, but they are not the same. Having taken an appropriate history, examined the patient and ordered any relevant investigations, the surgical nurse practitioners will then allow the patient to ask questions. Whatever information the patient requires will be given. The nurse practitioner can explain the surgical procedure, reassure the patient regarding anxieties, and discuss post-operative recovery with the patient and the patient's family. It is a fact that many patients still find doctors intimidating, and also that many doctors, despite changes in training, remain very poor listeners. The nurse practitioner will be asked far more questions than a medical

practitioner because patients don't feel a sense of inhibition with someone from a nursing background. The answers given by the nurse practitioner will probably also address issues a doctor wouldn't necessarily be involved with, and so be more helpful to the patient.

I am definitely not of the school of thought that regards the nurse practitioner as a doctor substitute. I do, however, believe that there are tasks traditionally carried out by doctors that can be performed by nurse practitioners, as well if not better than by the doctor. When performing the role of pre-operative assessment, the nurse practitioner takes a far more holistic approach to the patient than any junior doctor. This is not meant as a criticism of junior doctors – I was once a house officer myself, and my clerkings were as brief and narrowly focused as the very worst! For a junior doctor clerking a patient the focus is to get through it as quickly as possible, and preferably without a patient who asks questions, because there are always a hundred other things to do! A truly reprehensible attitude, but one that is a product of the workload.

Nurse practitioners are extremely versatile individuals who possess skills that will prove valuable wherever they work. They form a bridge between traditional nursing duties and traditional medical duties. In the pre-operative assessment setting the service benefits from consistence and reliability of patient assessment, leading to more efficient theatre time utilization. These benefits are possible because of the new skills and knowledge learned by the nurse practitioner. The patient benefits from less intimidating clerking, more time spent with them and far more information given. These benefits derive from the nurse practitioner's nursing background and skills. Whilst able to perform tasks previously viewed as medical, this is not a statement of intent. Rather, by performing these tasks nurse practitioners can free medical staff to devote extra time to more strictly medical duties.

I like to think that I am a forward-thinking doctor who focuses upon the patient and on teamwork. I believe that nurse practitioners form an important bridge between nursing and medical personnel and duties. The fears of nurses that the profession is moving away from core nursing values, and similarly the fears of doctors that nursing is eroding their clinical responsibilities, are fears borne out of paranoia. Nurses who want to be doctors leave nursing and become doctors. Nurse practitioners are here to prevent the two most important elements of health care delivery, the doctors and nurses, from drifting away from each other and pulling the poor patient in opposite directions. Nurse practitioners are here and, though I can foresee a few changes in title with time, they are here to stay. This is definitely good news for patients.

References

Arena, D. M. and Page, N. E. (1992). The imposter phenomenon in the clinical nurse specialist role. *J. Nursing Schol.*, **24(2)**, 121–5.

Benner, P. (1984). *From Novice to Expert: Excellence and Power in Clinical Nursing Practice*. Addison-Wesley.

Brown, M.-A. and Olshansky, E. F. (1997). From limbo to legitimacy: a theoretical model of the transition to the primary care nurse practitioner role. *Nursing Res.*, **46(1)**, 46–51.

Burke-Masters, B. (1986). The autonomous nurse practitioner: an answer to a chronic problem of primary care. *Lancet*, **1(8492)**, 1266.

Cable, S. (1994). What is a nurse practitioner? *Primary Health Care*, **4(5)**, 12–14.

Castledine, G. (1994). Specialist Nursing. An update on the UKCC's work into higher level practice. *British Journal of Nursing*, **3(12)**, 621–2.

Clance, P. R. and Imes, S. A. (1978). The imposter phenomenon in high achieving women: dynamics and therapeutic interventions. *Psychother: Theory, Res. Pract.*, **15**, 241–7.

Clay, T. (1991) The role of professional organisations. In: *Nurse Practitioners, Working for Change in Primary Healthcare Nursing* (J. Salvage, ed.), pp. 30–138. The King's Fund Centre.

Dimond, B. (1990). *Legal Aspects of Nursing*. Prentice-Hall.

Dreyfus, S. E. and Dreyfus, H. L. (1980). A five-stage model of the mental activities involved in directed skill acquisition. Unpublished report supported by the Air Force Office of Scientific Research (AFSC), USAF (Contract f49620-79-c-0063), University of California.

Emmerson, P. (1996). Are nurse practitioners merely substitute doctors? *Prof. Nurse*, **11(5)**.

Fawcett-Henesy, A. (1991). The British scene. In: *Nurse Practitioners, Working for Change in Primary Healthcare Nursing* (J. Salvage, ed.). The King's Fund Centre.

Ford, P. and Walsh, M. (1994). *New Rituals for Old: Nursing Through the Looking Glass*. Butterworth-Heinemann.

Hupcey, J. E. (1993). Factors and work settings that may influence nurse practitioner practice. *Nursing Outlook*, **41**, 181–5.

Loveland, P. (1992). The New Deal: an account of progress in reducing junior hospital doctors' hours in England. *Health Trends*, **24(1)**, 3–4.

National Health Service Management Executive (1991). *Junior Doctors: The New Deal*. NHSME.

Read, S. and Graves, K. (1994). *Reduction of Junior Doctors' Hours in Trent Region: The Nursing Contribution*. Trent Regional Health Authority.

Reveley, S. (1999). Introducing the nurse practitioner into general medical practice: operational and theoretical perspectives on the role. Unpublished PhD thesis, University of Lancaster.

Smith, G. and Cantley, C. (1985). *Assessing Health Care: A Study in Organisational Evaluation*. Open University Press.

Stilwell, B., Greenfield, S., Drury, V. W. M. and Hull, F. M. (1987). A nurse practitioner in general practice: working style and pattern of consultations. *J. R. Coll. GPs*, **37**, 1547.

United Kingdom Central Council for Nursing, Midwifery and Health Visiting (1992a). *The Scope of Professional Practice*. UKCC.

United Kingdom Central Council for Nursing, Midwifery and Health Visiting (1992b). *The Code of Professional Conduct for Nurses, Midwives and Health Visitors*. UKCC.

United Kingdom Central Council for Nursing, Midwifery and Health Visiting (1994). *Standards for Education and Practice following Registration*. UKCC.

Woods, L. (2000). *The Enigma of Advanced Nursing Practice*. Quay Books.

6

SETTING UP A NURSE PRACTITIONER-LED PRE-OPERATIVE ASSESSMENT CLINIC IN AN ORTHOPAEDIC UNIT

Shirley Reveley and Lesley Carruthers

Introduction

Pre-operative assessment clinics have emerged in response to an increased focus on improved patient care and cost constraints (Connaway and Blackledge, 1986; Takahashi and Bever, 1989). Orthopaedics was the first speciality to recognize the need for pre-assessment clinics, which date back to 1974 in the USA where the service was medically co-ordinated. In the UK the Duthie Report (DHSS, 1981) recommended pre-admission assessments for elective orthopaedic patients. In the hospital under discussion, prior to the introduction of nurse-led assessment clinics, patients were admitted to hospital the day before joint replacement surgery for laboratory tests, X-rays, medical consultation and nursing assessment. Treatment of identified health problems on admission often could not be completed before joint replacement surgery, resulting in cancellation of surgery. In addition, no formal education was given or occupational assessment undertaken regarding a patient's needs or home situation, which delayed the discharge planning requirements and prolonged the length of stay in hospital. Counsell and Gilbert (1999, p. 277) argue that advanced registered nurse practitioners have advanced training in the skills of assessment, diagnosis and treatment of medical and nursing conditions. In addition, they have strong decision-making skills and excellent skills in co-ordinating patient outcomes to provide quality cost-effective care:

They are becoming a mainstay practising in acute care settings, and hospitals are beginning to recognise their potential.

This chapter describes how a nurse practitioner was introduced into the orthopaedic unit of a district general hospital. The rationale for setting up the clinic, the barriers that the nurse practitioner encountered and how she overcame them are discussed, and the evaluation of the initiative is presented.

Finally, commentaries from a patient and an Acting Chief Executive regarding the nurse practitioner role in pre-operative assessment are included.

Setting up the clinic

The pre-operative assessment clinic was formally established in the orthopaedic unit of the district general hospital in 1995 following the appointment of a clinical nurse practitioner. The decision to establish a pre-operative assessment nurse practitioner-led clinic was reached by the business and ward managers, who had researched the benefits the nurse practitioner could bring to patient care. The aims of the pre-operative assessment clinic are to:

- Provide a complete physical, psychological, spiritual and social assessment of the patient
- Identify, treat and refer any needs or problems that could prevent any post-operative complications, delay or cancel the operation
- Facilitate the admission and discharge process
- Minimize the cancellation of patients for surgical intervention
- Maximize the use of bed management, organization of theatre nursing and medical time
- Benefit patients, ward and reduce waiting lists.

Pre-assessment covers the areas of autologus blood donation and patient education; it provides a forum for patients and family to discuss questions, share anxieties and concerns before the operation and hospitalization; it provides an holistic assessment from the nursing and medical staff, physiotherapist and occupational therapist; and it includes arranging laboratory tests; X-rays, and referral (if required) to another speciality.

Title of post: clinical nurse practitioner, orthopaedic service

Grade 2 Nurses & Midwives Trust Conditions, 37.5 hours per week. Responsible and accountable to Lead Consultant, Orthopaedics.

Job summary

To participate in a training/orientation and educational programme to enable the post-holder to be responsible for the care of inpatients and day cases registered under the consultant.

Key objectives of the role

1. *Clinical/professional*:
   - To practise in accordance with UKCC guidelines, the Medicines Act and the Ionising Radiation Regulations
   - To participate in elective pre-operative patient assessment, nursing assessment, history taking, and clinical examination of patients
   - To participate in the identification, resolution or referral of patients' undiagnosed problems to another speciality
   - To participate in follow-up clinics for patients who have undergone hip and knee surgery
   - In accordance with the protocol of nurse practitioner, orthopaedics, to request X-rays to ensure continuity of patient care
   - To perform practical procedures – phlebotomy, ECG, insertion of intravenous cannulae
   - To set standards of practice in conjunction with the ward manager
   - To participate in clinical audit as defined by the lead consultant and ward manager.
2. *Education and training*:
   - To act as an educational resource to staff by undertaking audit presentations and participating in training programmes.
3. *Communication*:
   - To liaise with appropriate ward managers and nursing teams for the treatment of

patients within the orthopaedic, short-stay and day-case areas
   - To develop a communication network that gains the maximum co-operation from personnel coming into contact with post-holder.

Main requirements for position

1. *Essential*:
   - First level general nurse
   - Minimum of 3 years' experience at Grade E/Trust 5 in orthopaedic- or intensive care-related nursing, but preferably to have practised at Grade F13
   - ENB 998 or City & Guilds 730
   - The post-holder must be willing to undertake a practitioner's qualification/degree.
2. *Desirable*:
   - First line management experience.

Appointing the clinical nurse practitioner

The decision to appoint a clinical nurse practitioner within the orthopaedic unit of the hospital NHS Trust was made by the business and ward managers resulting from the reduction in junior doctors' numbers by one under the New Deal (NHSME, 1991; Loveland, 1992), which set a limit to junior doctors' hours. Owing to the increasing workload and faster throughput of patients, the pressure on junior doctors is increasing. Such factors contributed to the reduction of time available to the patients, thereby creating a need to reconsider the workload of the junior doctors and identify those clinical tasks that could be accomplished by extending the role of the nurse.

Why a nurse practitioner rather than a clinical nurse specialist?

'Advanced nursing practice' is the term applied to those nurses who have acquired the knowledge and skills in speciality areas that allow the further expansion and advancement of the profession (Steel, 1997). Steel suggests that expansion means the acquisition of new skills for practice, whilst advancement of the nurse and the nursing profession occurs as a result of both specialization and expansion. She states that the roles of the nurse practitioner and the clinical nurse specialist complement each other and are both advanced nursing roles with many similarities between them. Nurse practitioners were formerly (in the USA) seen as experts in history taking and physical examination, the focus of their work being direct patients care. Clinical nurse specialists provided some direct care, but education, research and consultation were also parts of the role. Today both roles include all of these, but the difference is one of emphasis on different aspects. The nurse practitioner discussed in this chapter is involved largely in direct patient care, with some research and teaching in her work.

Furthermore, it has been argued that the nurse practitioner's skills are generic in scope and specialist in level, in terms of the United Kingdom Central Council's 1994 definition of specialist practice (Reveley, 1999). This perception is highlighted by the nurse practitioner in this extract from the interview:

> Well with a clinical nurse specialist in ortho-paedics, you're looking at that nurse being specialized in orthopaedics; with a nurse practi-tioner, you're looking more generic; a person who can look at the patient as a whole, not just the bone structure, not just the operation. Someone who can assess the patient, check medication, undertake a physical examination, document findings and look at the patient as a whole. Nurse specialists are very know-ledgeable in orthopaedics. They approach the patient from an orthopaedic point of view, not looking at any other problems the patient may have. I feel that the nurse specialist wouldn't be able to do what a nurse practitioner can for the patient, and that's assess the person holistically.

Before considering clinical practice as a clinical nurse practitioner within the ortho-paedic unit, it was necessary to establish what the job description/role of the senior nurse already in post entailed, alongside the job description for the clinical nurse practitioner. The senior nurse was responsible to the nurse ward manager, and the key areas of responsibility covered were service quality, organizational relationships, communication, management and finance. In comparison, the clinical nurse practitioner has responsibility and accountability to the lead consultant, and the key parts of the role are clinical/pro-fessional, educational, training and communi-cation.

Skill acquisition

The experience required by the Trust for the post of the clinical nurse practitioner role was acquired here through previous experience as a senior nurse, and a background of district nursing, hospice nursing, occupational health nursing and nursing in the acute care sector. Although the nurse did not have the necessary skills of history taking, co-ordinating the pre-assessment clinic, requesting X-rays, inserting i.v. cannulae, etc., her previous background and experience gave her the knowledge to commence a specific course of study – the BSc (Hons) Health Studies (Nurse Practitioner) programme. This resonates with Benner's (1984) position that:

> Strong educational preparation in the biological and psycho-social sciences and in the nursing arts and science is the necessary base for advanced skill acquisition, because this knowledge provides the basis for safe care.

In the early days of her nurse practitioner practice she was very dependent on the doctors:

> My role began for pre-assessment within the orthopaedic department – pre-assessment of joint replacement patients 2 weeks prior to surgery – and this was to do a full holistic assessment on them – to look at the medical, social aspects of the patient with regards to major surgery. It started initially very much from a nurse-based point of view because I didn't have the qualifications or the capability to be able to do this to the extent I'm actually doing it now. So I started off very much in a nurse role, and it was more a nursing assess-ment within a multidisciplinary team; physio-therapist, occupational therapist and the doctor. The doctor had quite a lot of input in the very early stages from the point of view of history taking, documentation, physical examination and investigations. I took the bloods, but the doctor got the results back and anything that needed to be done, he or she saw to this.

The nurse practitioner started with history taking at novice level, having had no experience of how to take a history or document the interaction. She had no understanding of how, why and when the questions to be asked should be posed, and how to analyse and evaluate the findings. The aim of history taking is to elicit an accurate account of the symptoms that represent the clinical problem and to set this against the background of the patient's life. Swash (1995) and Bates (1995) suggest that the interaction with a patient during history taking lays the foundation for good care. Until recently this has been the responsibility of the medical profession; nurses have taken a nursing assessment incorporating a history, but have not included the detailed clinical information taken by a doctor.

During the Role of the Nurse Practitioner Module, consultation style and documentation of history taking in the clinical area were taught by a general practitioner. Features of the task were given so that the importance of how the history taking was done and why were recognized. There was little opportunity to practise this in the orthopaedic unit, however, and therefore the nurse practitioner gained little understanding of the contextual meaning of the education. She therefore sought the help of medical and surgical facilitators, and attended the outpatient clinic with both facilitators to listen to and observe their consultations and gain situational experience.

Observing gave great insight into the technique and how a picture of the patient was to be developed, but the nurse practitioner was unable to perform these comprehensive tasks without prompts. She therefore developed a pro forma to help her take a detailed patient history. Consultations followed with both facilitators with regard to the pro forma content and permission to use it, as it was necessary to ensure there were no omissions that could give rise to complications for the patient.

The pro forma was very easy to use – it gave prompts and allowed no omissions – but it unfortunately provided no more than a tick list. This was adequate in assessing the patient, but prevented the development of history-taking skills. The pro forma was only allowing the nurse practitioner to detect the normal from the abnormal and to prioritize interventions.

The nurse practitioner gradually gained confidence:

An example of the development into competency was seeing my actions in terms of long-term goals. When a patient presents with hypertension at the pre-assessment clinic, with no previous history, this could be viewed as 'white-coat' hypertension and the pre-assessment could proceed. However, on admission into hospital the hypertension may remain, again as white-coat syndrome due to the anxiety of hospitalization or it may be clinical in origin. Whatever the reason for the hypertension the operation would be cancelled due to the risks of post-operative complications. Cancellation at such a late stage causes distress to the patient and family, inappropriate utilization of resources and an increase to the waiting lists. To avoid this situation the hypertension is addressed immediately by me referring the patient to their general practitioner for continual assessment monitoring or treatment to prevent a further cancellation of their operation.

When or how the nurse practitioner felt competent is not easy to say. After approximately 12 months she had the ability to take a full, detailed patient history without the use of prompts to link and understand the systems of life, to plan, to diagnose and identify problems, to make decisions and organize patient care. The proficient stage came very gradually. Learning from previous pre-assessments – analysing the situation and patient, the decision making, planning, admission care, the referral to other health care professionals and the co-ordination of patient care, and seeing the outcomes of pre-assessment in long-term goals – made the practice more effective for present and future patients. Gone were the tick box prompts with tasks to be undertaken for the operation to proceed; the stage arrived where the nurse practitioner assessed the patient holistically, gathering all the information to establish the situation as a whole and looking into long-term situations and not just the post-operative period:

As time went by as a nurse practitioner and I gained skills from the learning that I'd had from the physical examination, documentation, and communication from the course, eventually I developed the nurse practitioner role, which now doesn't have any doctor input unless I actually need it. If there's something wrong, that is when I bring the doctor in. I'm there to diagnose but not to do anything from there on. I bring the doctor in, but any of the correspondence with the patients, the communication with any other member of the multidisciplinary team, the anaesthetic department, the medical profession I do, not the junior doctor. It's just a matter of the seal of approval from the junior doctor, for example with heart murmurs or something like that.

Patient referral

When health problems are highlighted that could potentially cause post-operative complications, the patient requires referral to other specialists to prevent complications and ensure optimum health for the operation. The referrals could be to the patient's general practitioner, a specialist nurse in the acute care sector or primary care, or to a consultant within the hospital.

In the early stages, the nurse practitioner passed any health problems that required referral to the junior doctors. With time and practice and improvement in skills she began to reflect upon her practice, and realized that she was the person who was highlighting any potential health problems, making the decision for the referral and to which speciality. At the same time she was giving all the patient information to the junior doctor with the reason for the referral and suggesting to which person or department it had to go. She was also explaining the deferral of the operation to the patient, providing the junior doctor with the information to be put into the referral letter, and then the junior doctor gave the news to the patient as though it was his or her decision for the referral. The nurse practitioner was then left to counsel distraught patients who may have waited up to 12 months for this day only to be told that they were not medically fit for surgical intervention. This situation is resonant of the doctor–nurse game described by Stein (1967). In this situation the doctor orders treatment, but the treatment is based on the observation, knowledge and recommendation of the nurse practitioner.

The authority to carry out patient care is now in the domain of the nurse practitioner (Steel, 1997):

I questioned myself as to why I was allowing the doctors the authority to write the referral letter upon my recommendations, take the credit for preventing post-operative complications for the patient and improving the utilization of resources. After all, the only part the junior doctor was taking part in was the letter writing. Was it because in the past doctors always referred patients, or was I frightened of not having my referral accepted by the medical profession? For whatever reason, this practice had to stop. Reflecting upon my actions, the only part of the patient referral I was not undertaking was the writing of the referral letter. I therefore decided to take full responsibility to refer all patients to other specialities. To ensure good documentation was used I continued to use the medical referral letter for internal referrals and an open guide computer template for primary care. Both documents ensured accurate professional documentation.

Barriers to setting up the role

Some resistance came from nurses on the unit, and some from the anaesthetic department. There was also some resistance from another surgical unit. Part of this opposition was to do with the nurse practitioner being new to the unit and unknown to other health professionals. They questioned who she was, where she came from and what she knew. The nurse practitioner found it quite difficult in the very early stages.

Junior doctors and nurses

When the nurse practitioner was asked by her medical facilitator to go on the ward round in order to learn, the nurses on that ward were initially not very receptive to her. They questioned who she was, being allowed to go round all their patients on the ward rounds. What was she there for? What was her role? To overcome this she asked permission of the ward staff and explained why she wanted to accompany the consultant on the ward round.

The junior doctors didn't know what the role of the nurse practitioner was, but were interested and supportive:

> I would speak to the nurses before I would speak to the patient, then explain everything. Now the doctors were actually on board right away, they were very interested. Very eager to learn about the role and they could see where the role would help them along the way as well, I don't mean by being a doctor's handmaiden, but letting them treat the acutely ill patients and me the non-acute patients, and the senior house officers were very interested and they contributed well. I found the junior doctors and senior house officers from the medical wards accepted me a lot easier than did the nurses.

General practitioners

The hardest task was with the general practitioners; even with a personal telephone conversation and a computerized letter many were not prepared to accept the nurse practitioner's judgements and contacted the patient's consultant to dispute the referral. This made it very difficult for patients by prolonging the waiting time for admission into hospital, questioning the nurse practitioner's ability to assess patients, and preventing a good nurse–patient relationship. King (1991) suggests that in general practice opinions of nurse practitioners are, predictably, mixed, with some GPs believing them to be a threat to their role. This may explain the problems with GP acceptance of nurse practitioner referrals. Some GPs – those who don't see nurse practitioners as having a role – didn't feel that the nurse practitioner was the appropriate person to speak to. If she had any problems and rang them they asked to speak to the doctor, even though she was the one with the information. The junior doctors didn't have the information to give. When she began turning patients down for surgery, some GPs believed she was questioning whether they were monitoring their patients adequately:

> One GP complained to the Chief Executive and Director of Nursing about my practice, because I had turned five of his patients down. He asked who I was to turn down five of his patients at pre-op. assessment, and did I realize the confusion, the upset and everything that I have caused. The Director of Nursing came to see me and I proved, because I keep records of everything I do, I had evidence of why I'd turned them down. Two patients had diabetes, two were hypertensive, and one was actually in renal failure. Two of them had died. So I was left with three who couldn't be stabilized.

Loeffer (1994) states that patients will not benefit from conflict between the nursing and medical professions. This is true for patients of GPs disputing referrals from the nurse practitioner, because their wait for orthopaedic surgery was then increased. The situation had to be addressed to improve patient care. A meeting with the ward manager and the consultants was arranged to discuss why the GPs were not in agreement with her decisions, and perusal of the referred patients' notes was undertaken. Together with the findings from this process, and the rationale of her decisions, the consultants supported the nurse practitioner and confirmed this in writing to the GPs concerned. They also asked that the nurse practitioner's requests be addressed before they would proceed with patients' operations.

If the role of the nurse practitioner had been marketed better, there might not have been as much resistance and it may not have taken as long to be accepted into some of the GP practices. The nurse practitioner overcame a lot of problems by trying to communicate more effectively. She explained to all the practice receptionists who she was, what her role was and where she came from. She wrote to all the GPs so that they would be better informed, and also faxed them with information. Now that the nurse practitioner has spoken to many GPs on the telephone, has handled the situation carefully and explained exactly what she is expected to do and why, communication and relationships have improved.

Some GPs are undertaking good preoperative assessments on their patients, screening them for health problems so that operations are not cancelled unnecessarily. Some GP practices are now asking the nurse practitioner how they can assess their patients prior to surgery. She advises them to screen for infection, hypertension, diabetes, etc., and is finding that there is an improvement generally. This is very good for the patients waiting for operation.

Anaesthetists

At first the consultants in the anaesthetic department would contact the nurse practitioner by telephone and question some of her judgements. However, she was always well prepared, keeping accurate documentation at hand in order to answer any questions, ready to give her professional opinions and having any results from the investigations taken available. Her judgement was soon accepted, and there is now an excellent professional relationship.

Radiographers

During the Nurse Practitioner Module, education and training were given regarding ionizing radiation regulations and the safe assessment and management of patients requiring an X-ray. With the knowledge gained, which ensured safe practice for the patients and staff and allowed provision of a speedier and continuous service to the patients, a protocol was produced for the nurse practitioner in orthopaedics requesting radiographs. The nurse practitioner then approached the ward manager as to the feasibility of her being able to request X-rays for pre- and post-operative patients. She suggested that the nurse practitioner should contact the Head of Radiology.

The nurse practitioner thought that the best way was to approach the head radiographer, as support from him and his team would perhaps influence the radiologists to accept nurse practitioner requests. How wrong she was! She took the details of the education programme and the guidelines provided from the course to the head radiographer, only to be told that neither she nor any other ward nurse would ever be allowed to request X-rays when he and his own staff, with their greater knowledge of radiography, were unable to. He said that he had been trying to implement the requesting of X-rays by Accident and Emergency senior trained staff, but 12 months later had made no progress.

Deflated by this response and due to the pressures of work, the nurse practitioner allowed this issue to be put on hold, letting the doctors sign her X-ray requests. As she became more autonomous in the pre-assessment clinic, the only tasks she was asking the junior doctors for help with were X-ray referrals and the prescribing of drugs. This was preventing continuity of care for patients, who had to wait around until the doctor was available. Ironically, the doctors came to her for advice as to what examination was required.

This was hindering progress, so the nurse practitioner asked for a meeting with the ward manager and consultants to propose protocols to enable her to request X-rays. No problems could be foreseen and no objections were raised, so it was referred to the Clinical Policy Board Meeting with the hospital directors and radiologists. The outcome was that she was sanctioned to sign X-ray request forms on the understanding that her practice was audited. The nurse practitioner has now been requesting X-rays for a year, and there has been a great improvement in the quality of service being provided to the patients, carers, family, staff and the ambulance liaison service because of the reduction in waiting time. Patients using hospital transport can now have a booked time and be ready at their time of departure.

Enabling factors

Previous experience

Previous experience of working as a senior nurse and working with the consultants prior to taking up this post allowed good communication, as a rapport had developed between the nurse practitioner and consultants. The consultants also knew her level of competence in her previous role, which she believes made them feel that patients were 'safe' with her in relation to patient care. Thus the nurse practitioner had credibility, which helped to overcome any barriers there may have been.

Preparation of the environment

Hupcey (1993) asked nurses working in both primary and acute care about the workplace factors that supported or hindered their practice. Most frequently mentioned as an enabling factor was acceptance by doctors followed by support from co-workers. Negative factors included lack of understanding about the nurse practitioner roles, and the fear of encroaching on others' territory. Steel (1997) states that 'a great deal of education and information sharing must take place in the practice arena in order to prepare the environment for the arrival of the advanced registered nurse practitioner'. In the orthopaedic unit, open discussions and explanation were used to gain commitment to this new role among co-workers. There was initially some resistance to change, but now, 5 years later, there is reported to be total acceptance.

Managerial support

The clinical manager acted as mentor to the nurse practitioner, and this had a positive effect because the manager understood her needs, including educational and resource needs, and met them. This manager was committed to the role of the nurse practitioner and to the nurse practitioner herself. The business manager was also committed to this new development, and both these individuals were determined that it should work. The nurse manager encouraged the nurse practitioner to go to the various departments such as laboratories to explain who she was and what her role entailed. Staff appreciated this.

The medical facilitator

The nurse practitioner, medical facilitator and nurse manager worked together, the nurse manager from a nursing and resource perspective and the facilitator from an educational perspective. Having the commitment of a medical consultant was very important in enabling the nurse practitioner to develop assessment and history-taking skills. This facilitator was also a teacher of medical students, and had extensive experience of the needs of learners and assessment of their competence. As the nurse practitioner says:

> I feel I'm a very fortunate person because I've had their commitment – not just the commitment of, oh yes, I believe in nurse practitioners, but of their skills – from their skills and education, their understanding, they could put me on to the right path. This wasn't handed to me on a plate – I had to go and learn – but I was helped along the way with what books to read and their being interested as well. The facilitator would ask, 'How are you getting on? What don't you understand?' He talked me through, discussed things, and when I got frightened of ENT because I didn't do an awful lot of it he made an effort for me to be able to practise on the ward,

> he got me the equipment. He took me into his office, he educated me, showed me what to do, he was interested in what I found were problems. I went on his ward rounds, and this is where my teaching started. Now that was invaluable, excellent. He was teaching junior doctors and senior house officers at the time, so I had to sit in the background, because I didn't want to interfere with their teaching, but I learned so much from sitting in the background and all of a sudden I was joining in, and he included me. He never got me out of my depth, which I really appreciated.

Shah (1997) says that many physicians welcome the role of the nurse practitioner and become involved in teaching, mentoring and absorbing the new practitioner among the team. Trust and collaboration mark the working relationship, and the system benefits from physician colleagues. They need help, however, in understanding that 'nurse practitioners do not wish to take over their role but wish to practise to the fullest extent of their knowledge and profession' (Shah, 1997).

The junior doctors have accepted the nurse practitioner's role, not only because it lightens their workload but also because it enables team-working to in order get the work done and enhances the quality of patient care – as the following example shows:

> Four patients were admitted to the ward within 10 minutes of each other. The nurses were dealing with four patients who had suffered trauma. At the same time there were three patients being admitted for elective surgery. The junior doctor was on his own and he had no-one to rely on. The nurse practitioner therefore admitted the three elective patients whilst the doctor managed the acutely ill patients. All went smoothly and the doctor expressed his thanks to the nurse practitioner.

Autonomy

The nurse practitioner is now working at a high level of autonomy and decision making. She also participates in research and audit, including an international research project. She makes her own decisions as to whether a patient should or should not be admitted for elective surgery and relays this decision to the consultant. The following example illustrates the extent of this:

> A female patient came in who had urinary problems. From my examination and history taking I decided this was a not a gynaecological problem but an orthopaedic one. She couldn't get to the toilet in time and was slightly incontinent, so I let the patient come in and told the consultant what I thought. He asked whether I had examined the woman, which I had. He then said 'Do you feel this is a gynaecological problem?' and I said 'no'. The operation went ahead, and once she'd had a hip replacement she could get to the toilet. This consultant took my word. I'd made the decision, I'd worked on my own. When the patient had the operation, he said: 'Yes, you were right. You were completely right, it wasn't a gynaecological problem.'

Hicks and Hennessey (1999), from the results of their survey into defining the role of the nurse practitioner in acute and primary care, suggest that 'full autonomy for every stage of the patient's care is a priority for the acute sector nurse practitioner'. They also suggest that clinical examinations by acute sector nurse practitioners are by implication 'more critical and serious because a presenting primary problem has been identified to be of sufficient gravity to merit further hospital-based investigation'. They further suggest that these clinical examination skills might more rightly be in the medical than the nursing domain.

The nurse practitioner has demonstrated that she is competent to make an assessment of a patient's health status, detect deviations from the norm, and act on the basis of her findings. However, this decision making takes place within an ethical/legal framework. She also works within a frame of practice agreed by the hospital Trust. She works to a protocol for transcribing previously prescribed medication, and a protocol for prescribing radiographs.

Improving the service

The pre-operative assessment clinic is now not only for patients requiring joint replacement but also for patients requiring intermediate and day surgery. Any patient with medical problems sees the nurse practitioner 2 weeks before admission. The patients report that they feel they are getting a good MOT, as they call it, and they also feel valued. They are also coming in prepared for surgery:

> I do a nursing assessment, a physical assessment, medical documentation, investigations, education, communication with the social work department if necessary. I actually look at the social aspects of patients' lives because they may be caring for somebody in their own home and they're frightened how these people are going to manage. So these patients feel that they're being treated as a whole person and I communicate with the occupational therapy department and physiotherapy. I feel that the patients are being given an holistic assessment, not just a nursing assessment, a medical assessment or whatever you'd like to call it. That's how I feel the nurse practitioner role has taken over now.

Traditionally in acute hospitals patient care has been managed by doctors and delivered by nurses, doctors and various other health professionals who perform their own assessments and develop their own plans of care (Steel, 1997). The nurse practitioner can offer a global perspective on patient care through the nursing process and, because she combines an advanced level of clinical expertise with interpersonal skills and blends nursing and medical skills, is ideally placed to provide holistic care (Steel, 1997).

A care pathway approach has been introduced into the orthopaedic unit, and this involves all the multidisciplinary team. The patients have ownership of their treatment plan and are partners in care; they know exactly what to expect. The patients feel very good about this because they know they are part of this assessment – they are not just being assessed, they can contribute. After 6 years the pre-assessment clinic is well established and people know how to contact the nurse practitioner. The patients have contact telephone numbers and can contact the nurse practitioner 3 months after the operation to see if things are going right, or to ask for advice. Patients are not forgotten when they go out; they can ring up for advice after the pre-op. assessment. They can also ring up before they come in, so the patients are very much involved in their rehabilitation. Steel (1997) also stresses the importance of this, arguing that in the current medical structure doctors are not as readily available as nurses. The nurse practitioner can be available to the patient and family even after discharge, and they are able to telephone regarding any concerns. The nurse practitioner, Steel suggests, combines nursing and medical information to meet patient and family needs.

Gradual acceptance of the role and of her abilities by other health care professionals has made for a more effective and efficient service for patients. In the past many patients lost their ambulance 'pick up' slot whilst waiting for a doctor. This sometimes delayed them for 2 hours or more, causing huge problems and anxiety for the ambulance liaison service, patients, their families and carers. The patients waiting for their post-operative check X-ray can now have the X-ray request in the X-ray department first thing in the morning. The patient is taken to the department and the films are available for the consultant's 11 o'clock ward round, and mobilization can commence the first day post-operatively. In the past X-ray request forms were frequently not signed until after the consultant's ward round, and the patient had to remain on bed rest until the following day when the X-rays were seen by the consultant and mobilization was allowed to commence. The patients are now getting a better service.

Cost-effectiveness

Nurse practitioners in the USA have been shown to deliver cost-effective care (Counsell and Gilbert, 1999). In the UK it has been argued that care provided by nurse practitioners may be no cheaper than care provided by doctors. This has been linked to the longer consultation times of nurse practitioners (Salisbury and Tettersell, 1988; Reveley, 1998). There is much evidence to demonstrate that nurse practitioners can reduce waiting times for patients whilst also increasing patient satisfaction (Marshall, 1997; Reveley, 1998). Hicks and Hennessey (1999) suggest that:

The unassailability of these arguments, coupled with the cogent empirical evidence thus far amassed both nationally and internationally, would indicate that the NP is a valid means by which high quality health care could be provided within stringent budgetary restrictions.

An audit of the pre-operative assessment clinic in this orthopaedic unit was undertaken over an 18-month period. Out of a total of 700 patients attending the pre-operative assessment clinic over this time, 155 were referred, deferred or cancelled; 144 of these patients were for joint replacement surgery. Had these patients been admitted for surgery the day before operation, as would have happened prior to the nurse practitioner assessing them 2 weeks before admission, the cost to the Trust of operations cancelled on the day of surgery would have been substantial. To assess what this cost might have been, an estimation was made based on giving the 144 patients an average stay of 8.5 days at £150 per day – a total of £183 600 – plus theatre sessions of 3 hours per patient, costing £181 440 altogether. The saving to the Trust was therefore estimated to be (£365,040).

All patients attending the orthopaedic clinic who are placed on the waiting list for surgery are entered onto a waiting list pro forma by a doctor. The intention is to identify patients' underlying medical conditions and to refer patients to the pre-operative assessment clinic. The pre-operative assessment clinic has been very successful in screening patients undergoing major surgery and those identified with potential problems on the waiting list pro forma. Despite the introduction of the waiting list pro forma and the pre-operative assessment clinic, theatre cancellations are still occurring within 24 hours of the planned operation. In an attempt to reduce the number of such cancellations, the following measures have been introduced:

1. Patients are asked to confirm their place on the operation list
2. Postal questionnaires are sent out to patients 2 months prior to surgery to identify medical problems, medical conditions that have been diagnosed after the patient was placed on the waiting list, and social factors that might prevent patients attending for surgery.

The results of the questionnaires are vetted by the ward manager, and all patients with identified medical problems are assessed by the nurse practitioner.

Patient satisfaction

Over a 5-month period from December 1996 to April 1997, 50 patients were asked to complete a patient satisfaction questionnaire in order to evaluate their perceptions and expectations of the pre-operative assessment clinic. The process was repeated from September 1997 to February 1998. Response rates were high; 82 per cent in the first survey, and 92 per cent in the second. All had been seen by the nurse practitioner. All respondents stated they had been given the opportunity to ask questions. Over 50 per cent had been introduced to the orthopaedic team, 95 per cent had been satisfied with the information/ education they had received, all had been given a contact telephone number, and 90 per cent were fully satisfied with their experience at the clinic.

It is acknowledged that, in general, patient satisfaction surveys consistently yield high satisfaction with care. However, this is no reason not to conduct them (Vuori, 1991). The patient satisfaction surveys and the audits that have taken place are testimony to the ongoing success of this particular pre-operative assessment clinic.

Conclusion

Assessment of patients 2 weeks prior to joint replacement provides:

- An holistic assessment by the multidisciplinary team
- Diagnostic tests
- An improvement in the discharge process by identifying potential problems and patient needs that can be addressed prior to admission
- Identification, resolution or referral of the patient with undiagnosed medical problems in the pre-operative stage in order to prevent post-operative complications
- Time for a pre-operative education programme for patients and their relatives to share anxieties, ask questions and discuss their concerns before admission to hospital
- The opportunity to be assessed within the surroundings in which they will be cared for during and after their surgery, thus allowing them to familiarize themselves with the ward and the staff who will be caring for them.

The above factors result in increased satisfaction among patients, meet patients needs in a proactive manner, constitute an holistic approach to care, and are a means of containing costs through more efficient use of resources.

Maskell and Wright (1993) found that the combination of assessment and education pre-operatively resulted in a significant decrease in orthopaedic surgery cancellations, decreased the length of hospital stay and allowed comprehensive discharge planning, and that the patients' experience was more positive. However, Shah (1997) comments that hospitals will have to commit to the concept of nurse practitioners. This commitment takes many forms:

1. *Respect* for the nursing profession in ways that have not always been historically obvious or prominent
2. *Protection* for the practitioner, with streamlined system policies that facilitate credentialling and suitably guard against unwarranted legal intrusion
3. *Nurturance* for the new role by establishing realistic expectations regarding the scope and breadth of practice responsibilities
4. *Compensation* for nurse practitioners that reflects the increased level of responsibilities and advanced practice skills they bring to patient care.

The nurse practitioner discussed in this chapter does have the support and respect of her colleagues such that at the level of the individual hospital or unit the role can be seen to be valued. What Shah (1997) is asking for is actually needed at a higher level than the hospital; respect, protection, nurturance and compensation must come from the profession of nursing itself, and nursing's statutory body must take the lead.

A patient's commentary on the nurse practitioner role in pre-operative assessment

The following commentary comes from an 80-year-old male patient:

I met this nurse practitioner a year ago when I came to the hospital to be assessed for an operation on my ankle. I also had a problem with my knee. She assessed me to see if I was fit for an operation at my age. Anyway, the operation didn't happen at that time for other reasons.

I had an idea what a nurse practitioner was from what other people had said, like health promotion. I take an interest, you know, and I came to see the nurse practitioner again a week before my operation this year. She assessed me and I thought it was a good idea. I didn't realize what went on properly until then. When you had to come to the hospital for operations before, they used to bring you up the day before and if you weren't fit they would send you home the day before your operation. I suppose that last year I spoke to the nurse practitioner about my operation because I thought the surgeon was elsewhere. I knew what the nurse practitioner was doing had always been done by a doctor, and the first time I came up to see this nurse practitioner over a year ago, I was a bit surprised at what did happen, seeing the nurse practitioner not the doctor.

When I came to see her this time I knew what to expect. She did a full physical examination and took a complete history, all about me. I got a bit upset because since I had come last time I had lost my wife, who had been very ill. The nurse practitioner said, 'it's all right to be upset', and we talked about it and about a bereavement she had had recently. I talked about my wife's illness and about her hospital stay, and the nurse practitioner really listened and was sympathetic. No one had done that before. Then I was sent off to get my bloods tested and everything and it was all done in one day.

I think the nurse practitioner is a good idea and I think nurses should be used more. I think that the better nurses are trained, the better it is for the health service, which really has been absolutely ravaged.

An Acting Chief Executive's commentary on the nurse practitioner role in pre-operative assessment

[The following commentary comes from Brian Earley, Acting Chief Executive of West Cumbria Health Care Trust, West Cumberland Hospital, Whitehaven, Cumbria]

It will come as no surprise to anyone involved in health care generally, and to those working in acute surgery particularly, that the vexed question of late cancellations of patients due to changes in their clinical condition which have not been picked up causes immense dissatisfaction, confusion and upset to the patients. It creates extra work for staff on the wards and makes the meeting of any pre-set targets for elective surgery difficult, if not impossible. Taken from the patients' perspective, it is extremely difficult for them to understand that they can be seen by a GP and by a consultant in a clinic and be referred for further surgery, and yet when they arrive no one is aware that there has been a change in their clinical condition that makes surgery inappropriate or more risky than they had been led to believe. It is very easy to underestimate the trauma that these individual patients go through when they have built themselves up for what could be major surgery and made social arrangements, only to be told at the very last moment, often on the day of surgery, that this cannot be carried out and that they will need to be assessed again.

We decided to look at orthopaedics specifically as, in common with other units nationally, we have considerable waiting lists and the time intervals between being seen in the outpatient clinic and arriving on the ward are sufficient to allow clinical changes to occur. Until there are sufficient orthopaedic surgeons, beds, nurses and theatre space to shorten the interval between initial assessment and admission drastically, we need to have a workable system which will ensure that patients are fully assessed much nearer to the time of admission, looking at their total health and not merely whether or not they need the orthopaedic procedure. Over the hill like the cavalry at the last moment comes the nurse practitioner!

Since the inception of the nurse practitioner pre-assessment clinic, my belief is that it has been tremendously successful; the numbers of patients cancelled on the day of surgery have dropped to virtually nil. Patients' satisfaction with the service is extremely high, and the doctors now accept, almost without conflict, the decision to defer any individual patients. They now accept that the nurse practitioner degree and the qualities of the individual concerned mean that any decision she makes is well-founded, and is reached on the basis of a sound clinical knowledge and a breadth of experience in orthopaedics and general nursing.

From a purely management point of view it

has certainly helped to maintain our patient throughput, and it is something that I would plan to extend to other areas of elective surgery, as we now have a track record of demonstrable improvement that has led to increased patient satisfaction and efficiency for the orthopaedic service.

References

Bates, B. (1995). *A Guide to Physical Examination and History Taking*, 6th edn. Lippincott.

Benner, P. (1984). *From Novice to Expert*. Addison-Wesley.

Connaway, C. A. and Blackledge, D. (1986). Pre-operative testing centre. *AORN J.*, **43(3)**, 666–70.

Counsell, C. and Gilbert, M. (1999). Implementation of a nurse practitioner role in an acute care setting. *Crit. Care Nursing Clin. North Am.*, **11(2)**, 277–82.

DHSS (1981). Orthopaedic Services: Waiting Times for Outpatient Appointments and Inpatient Treatments (Duthie Report), London: HMSO.

Hicks, C. and Hennessey, D. (1999). A task-based approach to defining the role of the nurse practitioner: the views of UK acute and primary sector nurses. *J. Adv. Nursing*, **20(3)**, 666–73.

Hupcey, J. E. (1993). Factors and work settings that may influence nurse practitioner practice. *Nursing Outlook*, **41**, 181–5.

King, R. (1991). Medical perspectives. In: *Nurse Practitioners Working for Change in Primary Health Care Nursing* (J. Salvage, ed.). King's Fund Centre.

Loeffer, A. S. (1994). Health care reform. Extending the role of nurse practitioners. *P.A. Nurse*, **49(7)**, 7.

Loveland, P. (1992). The New Deal: an account of progress in reducing junior hospital doctors' hours in England. *Health Trends*, **24(1)**, 3–4.

Marshall, J. (1997). Protocols and emergency nurse practitioners. *Nursing Times*, **93(14)**, 58–9.

Maskell, M. and Wright, J. (1993). Pre-operative preparation for patients undergoing total joint replacement. *CONA*, **15**, 112–15.

National Health Service Management Executive (1991). *Junior Doctors – the New Deal*. London.

Nolan *et al.* (1997).

Reveley, S. (1998). The role of the triage nurse practitioner in general medical practice: an analysis of the role. *J. Adv. Nursing*, **28(3)**, 584–91.

Reveley, S. (1999). Introducing the nurse practitioner into a group general medical practice: operational and theoretical perspectives on the role. Unpublished PhD thesis, University of Lancaster.

Salisbury, C. J. and Tettersell, M. (1988). Comparison of the work of a nurse practitioner with that of a general practitioner. *J. R. Coll. GPs*, **38**, 314–16.

Shah, S. S. (1997). Acquiring clinical skills and integrating them into the practice setting. In: *The Acute Care Nurse Practitioner* (B. J. Daly, ed.), p. 107. Springer Publishing.

Steel, J. E. (1997). Development of the acute nurse practitioner role: questions, opinions, consensus. In: *The Acute Care Nurse Practitioner* (B. J. Daly, ed.), pp. 21–47, 278–80. Springer Publishing.

Stein, L. (1967). The doctor–nurse game. *Arch. Gen. Psychiatry*, **16**, 699–703.

Swash, M. (1995). *Clinical Methods*. Saunders.

Takahashi, J. J. and Bever, S. C. (1989). Pre-operative nursing assessments. *AORN Journal*, **50(50)**, 1022–35.

United Kingdom Central Council for Nursing, Midwifery and Health Visiting (1994). *Standards for Education and Practice following Registration*. UKCC.

Vuori, H. (1991). Patient satisfaction – does it matter? *Qual. Assurance Health Care*, **3(3)**, 183–9.

7

THE DEVELOPING ROLE OF PAEDIATRIC NURSE PRACTITIONERS IN THE HOSPITAL SETTING: PLANS AND EMERGING ISSUES

Fiona Smart

Introduction

Roles develop in the provision of health care for a reason. This was the case in the nineteenth century, when the advancement of medicine required the services of a skilled workforce to care for the patients, and it is still the case now. As Doyal and Cameron (2000) observe, the traditional map of health care provision is being redrawn in response to circumstances that demand change. The way that it seems always to have been, will be no more. Walsh (2000) agrees, but adds that the motive underpinning change should concern only one reason; the best interests of the patient. Change that promotes the interests of professional groups, service managers or policy makers is therefore not appropriate. However, it might be that, as a consequence of putting patients first, gains ripple out to impact on others. Equally, it is possible that what some see as a gain represents a loss to others. Change is a complex phenomenon, and it may not be possible to predict winners and losers. Nevertheless, central to the concerns of the change-makers must the lie the interests of patients. If they do not stand to gain from the change proposed, its implementation should be questioned.

This chapter explores the early days of the introduction of a paediatric nurse practitioner role to the children's ward in two small district general hospitals in the north of England. The background to the role's development will be presented, along with issues emerging as a consequence of its introduction. Particular attention will be paid to the construction of the role and its potential to benefit children and families. However, it will also become apparent that although the paediatric nurse practitioner role is seen by some as an opportunity for the service to develop around the needs of children and their families, others see it differently. There is a reason why the role is developing,

but it is not universally welcomed. One issue of note is whether the paediatric nurse practitioner role belongs to children's nursing, or sits outside its sphere of practice. This will be argued to be a critical issue with consequences for children's nursing and its professional development.

The chapter is written through the eyes of an educationalist but its perspective is professional, reflecting a children's nursing background of some 20 years' standing. Service managers may well see the role and its development from another angle, as may colleagues from a medical background. The chapter draws on a substantial body of literature emerging from both the UK and the USA. It is also enriched by understandings that are developing as a result of researching the paediatric nurse practitioner role as it emerges over time in the two local settings. Data from this MPhil/PhD study are presented as part of this chapter and are drawn from interviews carried out with 26 participants (22 health care providers and four paediatric nurse practitioner students) on the two sites in 1999/2000, when the paediatric nurse practitioner initiative was in its very early stages.

The chapter is completed by a commentary by an American paediatric nurse practitioner lecturer.

Circumstances supporting the emergence of the paediatric nurse practitioner role

Ford's (1997) analysis of the development of the nurse practitioner movement in the USA in the 1960s directs attention to multiple forces that converged to create the opportunity for the role to emerge. She identifies three forces, social, political and professional; all three were necessary to the subsequent proliferation of nurse practitioner roles in a range of primary care settings. Citing a meta-analysis undertaken in 1986 by the Office of Technology Assessment, Ford (1997) notes that within their areas of competence nurse practitioners demonstrated that the quality of their care was equal to that of physicians. Moreover, they were found to be more adept at providing services requiring communication with patients or preventive action. Nurse practitioners met patients' needs; even more importantly, their contribution was cost effective (Brush and Capezuti, 1996).

In the 1990s, Knaus et al. (1997) wrote that nurse practitioners in the USA were presented with 'compelling opportunities' to take the role into the hospital setting. Once again, social, political and professional factors were converging to create demand for alternative models of care provision that were not dependent on medical practitioners (Ford, 1997). The need to contain cost but still provide a quality of service to an ever more demanding public was paramount (Brush and Capezuti, 1996; Knaus et al., 1997; Miller, 1998). Nurse practitioners were identified as care providers who could meet the need (Knaus et al., 1997).

So social, political and professional factors converged in the USA to create the circumstances within which the nurse practitioner movement could develop in primary, acute and critical care settings (Ford, 1997). Although health care systems are different in the UK, it seems that similar agendas are important here too, namely those of the government, consumers, the professions and service managers. Thus, the nurse practitioner role can be seen as developing in response to a unique combination of converging agendas, with time and place acting to enable its beginnings.

Imagine a window with the four agendas, one at each corner. Although separately, each is important in its own way, none on its own creates quite the same opportunities for re-organizing health care provision. It is in their interrelationships that change becomes possible and the window starts to bulge open. For example, although the government looks to a transformed health service 'redesigned around the needs of its patients' (Milburn, DoH, 2000), it knows that it depends on professional groups if the vision is to be

realized (DoH, 2000). Furthermore, it seems that in developing its plan for reform of the NHS, the government was influenced by a consumerist movement that is aware of its rights and is asserting them (Hutton, 2000).

This said, although all four agendas are claimed to be integral to the process creating the opportunity for change, it is not argued that there has to be a particular sequence of events. Change might be government driven, consumer led, professionally orchestrated or a service initiative. What is contended is that for it to happen, the change needs to be supported by all four corners of the window. If not, it cannot fully open to the opportunity afforded by change. This contention is now illustrated in the following case study of local change that has resulted in the development of a paediatric nurse practitioner role.

Local circumstances and change

Almost 2 years before the government published its plan for reform of the NHS (DoH, 2000), in a move that can be seen as proactive a local Health Authority commissioned a review of its paediatric services across community and hospital-based settings. Numerous recommendations were made; many were innocuous, but one was not. The review looked at inpatient children's services and devised four options for change. One option proposed the closure of one children's ward in order to consolidate services at the other site. The reasons behind the proposal of this option were complex, but were in part a response to existing and future problems with medical cover. The option was reported in the press and resulted in the presentation of a 32 000-name petition to the Health Authority. Parents wanted their local inpatient children's ward kept open. They knew that although the other children's ward was only 40 miles away, it took at least an hour to travel the distance. They saw this journey as potentially detrimental to their children's health.

The Health Authority's task force set up to deliberate on the findings of the review elected not to pursue the 'closure' option. Instead it decided to maintain inpatient services on both sites, but explore alternatives to the current model of service provision that relied on junior doctors who were often inexperienced and needed to be supported by consultant paedi-atricians. The 6-monthly rotation of junior doctors intensified this need for back-up at particular points in the year, and was seen as impacting negatively on current senior medical staff and the potential to recruit new con-sultants.

Exploring its options, the task force's attention fell on another of the review's recommendations. The review had suggested that a paediatric nurse practitioner role could be developed to 'support non-acute paediatric care and reduce the workload of the con-sultants'. The nature and scope of this role was not explored further in the document. How-ever, the task force picked the idea up and developed it into something that envisaged the paediatric nurse practitioner in a 'front-line' role. In effect, the task force sought paediatric nurse practitioners who would be able to assess children on admission to the ward and initiate the management of their presenting problem as appropriate. It was to be more than a triage role, and was to draw in the skills of history taking and physical examination. It was thought that the role would enable the inpatient services on both sites to be main-tained. In addition, it was seen that it would orientate the service away from reliance on junior doctors, who were in the main inexperi-enced and transient, and enable provision to develop using staff who were more attuned to children and families and far more permanent. It was a role to be invested in because of what the task force saw it could achieve in time. It was, however, a long-term solution to a press-ing problem. It was estimated that it would take a minimum of 3 years to prepare a paediatric nurse practitioner for practice, and probably closer to 6 years for the six paediatric nurse practitioners planned for each site to be established in their roles and for the service to be enhanced around children's and families' needs. This was no quick fix, although as a plan it progressed at some speed.

The task force presented its report in March 1999. By November 1999, a new route through an existing well-regarded nurse practi-tioner course at the local higher education institution had been validated. Three students began their part-time studies in January 2000. They are scheduled to complete in 2003, ready to take up their paediatric nurse practitioner roles in practice. In addition to these three

students, a graduate from the local nurse practitioner programme who is a children's nurse was recruited to undertake the double module focused on developing as a paediatric nurse practitioner alongside the three other students. The intention is that these four individuals will begin the process of enhancing the hospital-based service that is currently available to children and families. The task force also acknowledged that the paediatric nurse practitioner initiative was in line with the development of nursing roles into areas of practice previously not part of their remit. In short, the introduction of the role was perceived to be beneficial to the service users, service providers and the service itself. When the government published its plan for reform of the NHS in July 2000, it was clear that the role envisaged for the children's wards on the two sites was congruent with its thinking too. The window to change opened.

Nevertheless, issues have emerged in the wake of decision to run with the paediatric nurse practitioner option. The intention is to explore some of these here, especially those that add to the debate regarding the nurse practitioner/paediatric nurse practitioner role. In particular, attention will be given to competing constructions of the paediatric nurse practitioner role in the local settings and their potential to impact on the service users, its providers and the service itself. Focus will fall on the question of whether the paediatric nurse practitioner role belongs to children's nursing or not. In addition, some of the practicalities concerning the preparation of student paediatric nurse practitioners for practice will be addressed. It is important to note that minimal space will be afforded to what might be regarded as the 'big issues' – for example, the debate regarding the UKCC's position on nurse practitioner roles, especially its decision not to protect the title. This is explored in depth in Chapter 3. Discussion concerning issues related to the law and professional accountability will also not feature. Readers are advised to access Reveley (1999) for an analysis of the position as it relates to nurse practitioner roles.

The role as planned

The paediatric nurse practitioner role is not

new in the UK. Kobryn and Pearce (1991) reported the introduction of a paediatric nurse practitioner initiative in an Accident and Emergency department, developed to reduce waiting times. Callaghan *et al.* (1997) wrote of a paediatric nurse practitioner role in paediatric day care, and identified the role as centred on preparing the child and family for interventions, co-ordinating care, supporting the family and ensuring that follow-up is organized. Dearmun and Gordon (1999) reported on a paediatric nurse practitioner role set up in paediatric ambulatory care that involved history taking, clinical assessment, requesting X-rays and carrying out cannulation. In common, all three roles sought to enhance children's and families' experiences of health care; however, they differ one from another in the focus of their activities. There is nothing unusual about this; indeed Woods (1999) would argue that this is to be expected. Advanced nursing roles develop to meet local needs and are contingent on the setting (Woods, 1999).

The role identified for the two local settings featured in this chapter is different again. However, what makes it different can also be seen as making the role contentious and controversial. Unlike the role presented by Kobryn and Pearce (1991), which limited its scope of practice to children over 1 year of age with minor injuries (therefore medical or surgical emergencies were not part of the remit, and neither were children with head injuries), paediatric nurse practitioners in the role envisaged for these two settings will deal with whatever comes through the door. This said, it might be that 'dealing with' involves an immediate referral to a medical colleague. Children of any age and with any presenting problem will be the focus of the paediatric nurse practitioner's work. Where appropriate, the expectation is that the paediatric nurse practitioners will be able to gather sufficient data from the history and the physical examination to make a differential diagnosis and initiate treatment. Consequently, the paediatric nurse practitioner role planned for the two settings can be seen as taking the practitioners to the heart of medical territory. Davison (Dickson, 1996) and Hughes (1998), among others, maintain that diagnosis and treatment lie central to the practice of being a doctor.

Data from MPhil/PhD studies suggest that some participants are wholly positive about the development of the paediatric nurse practitioner role as planned. It is viewed as enhancing the service offered to children and their families because it utilizes the skills of experienced children's nurses in order to meet their needs. Some participants also see the role as impacting positively on children's nursing itself, because it offers a way forward for its practitioners that is clinically based. However, the role as planned can also be seen to generate concerns. Three are now featured; each relates to the other and is part of a picture of uncertainty that is balanced by a belief that children and families will gain from this initiative. The first two issues are closely linked, and relate to a perception that paediatric nurse practitioners might not be prepared for practice.

Prepared for practice?

The first issue concerns the preparation of paediatric nurse practitioners for practice, and raises questions as to whether they will be fit for purpose. Opinions vary. Some participants in the study point to medicine's knowledge base. Not only it is recognized as being broader, but also medical students are prepared over a longer period of time and consequently they are seen to know more. Yet it is also evident in the data that junior doctors on 6-monthly rotations through paediatric settings are seen to be limited in their capacity to use their knowledge base. It was not uncommon for participants in the study to talk about experienced children's nurses guiding junior doctors in their decision making; yet this was not seen to be the same as children's nurses actually making the decision themselves.

So junior doctors were recognized by participants as limited in their ability to practice in the paediatric setting, especially early on in a 6-month rotation. In contrast, participants saw experienced children's nurses as being skilled not only in working with children and families, but also in their capacity to identify a sick child who needs intervention. However, although experienced children's nurses are valued for this skill, some participants questioned whether it is underpinned by knowledge. As one person put it, they may know, but do not know why. It is not an unusual proposition. Calkin (1984) explored it at length in her model for advanced nursing practice, and spoke about 'experts by experience'. In short, experienced children's nurses have skills beyond their knowledge base, whereas junior doctors might be likened to novices whose knowledge runs ahead of their skills base.

From an educational perspective, Calkin's (1984) model provides direction. If experienced children's nurses understand children and families and are skilled in working with them, what they need for paediatric nurse practitioner practice is a knowledge base to underpin their practice and enable them to move into the field of diagnostic reasoning and clinical decision making. This will be facilitated for the three students recruited in January 2000 by a 3-year part-time course that requires academic development and its application to practice. Crumbie talks more about the rigours of the course of preparation in Chapter 9. However, it is worth mentioning here that, in recognition of the broad field of practice that will be the paediatric nurse practitioners' domain, particular attention is paid in the curriculum to commonly presenting symptoms. It is these that the students will learn to work with and connect together to make their diagnoses and decide on their management plan. In the early stages of their practice, anything that falls outside 'the common' will demand medical back-up. In effect, this puts a safety net in place until such time as they are able to work with a broader and broader range of presenting symptoms.

However, whether paediatric nurse practitioners will be educationally prepared for practice was seen in the data to be less of an issue than whether they will be able accept the responsibility and risk that comes with diagnosis and treatment. It is not that the paediatric nurse practitioner will suddenly be exposed to responsibility and risk – both are inherent in everyday practice – but, as Reveley (1999) acknowledges, the nurse practitioner may feel more exposed and vulnerable on the edge of the boundary of nursing practice. However, Annandale and Clark (1996) explain that a role focused on diagnosis and treatment will invoke more risk. Citing Paget (1988),

they write:

Signs and symptoms do not order themselves into neat diagnostic categories, nor do they unequivocally signal the 'correct' treatment regimen. Rather the process of acquiring, interpreting, managing and reporting the disorders of human illness is an error-ridden process.

Paediatric nurse practitioners in these two local settings will enter this world of uncertainty. The increased potential for error may be very stressful for them. There is an argument in the literature supported by data from the MPhil/PhD study that dealing with risk is a more accepted feature of medical practice and one from which nurses have been shielded in the past by the nature of their roles. However, expanded roles for nursing can be seen as pushing the boundaries and taking nurses into new territory where they may have to deal with new pressures, or old pressures experienced in a new way. The paediatric nurse practitioner role planned for these two settings is an example of that. Diagnosis and treatment have not been associated with the nursing role, but for Annandale and Clark (1996; citing Paget, 1988) entry into this territory will incur risk and might heighten perceptions of vulnerability.

One participant in the MPhil/PhD study spoke eloquently about the difficulties that will be faced by paediatric nurse practitioners. In doing so, it becomes evident that medical practitioners do not deal easily with the pressure either:

I think there are difficulties for the individual paediatric nurse practitioner, one of which is going to be loneliness. It's very lonely in the middle of the night, even after [x] years in paediatrics. I feel very lonely sometimes, in the middle of the night when I realize there's nobody else. ... I think that's something that we're going to have to build into their training. How to handle the fact that you've just failed, because they will fail, we all have. We all make mistakes. ... They're going to have demands on them that they've not experienced before and they're going to fail in a way that probably they've never failed before, especially if it results in a death. ... If a child dies they will probably feel they've failed, even it they didn't. If it was nothing to do with them, but you always feel that maybe there was something you could have done and I don't think they'll ever have experienced that. ...

Another participant adds a further dimension to this, speaking about what it is that makes medicine difficult:

As a doctor you are told to use your common sense and make decisions in the light of inadequate information. You know, you have to take risks really because you don't have all the facts. It's making decisions in the light of inadequate information. ... It is often the case in medicine that one only has half the jigsaw and has to guess the rest. The downside can be a tendency to cut corners – for example, getting a quarter of the jigsaw and not bothering to get the other quarter before making the guess.

Interestingly, rather than seeing that having to operate in the light of inadequate information would trip up paediatric nurse practitioners, this participant thought that their background as nurses would equip them to deal with it. This is explained on the basis of nurses' tendency to be rule followers rather than risk takers. Consequently, they would be less likely to cut corners and make unnecessary mistakes. Davies (2000) would question this. For him, nurses' rule-bound backgrounds do not easily prepare them for nurse practitioner roles.

It is probably the case that, for the two local settings, time will tell. However, to date, evidence in the literature in respect of other nurse practitioner roles does not suggest that they cannot deal with risk in practice. That said, the paediatric setting might be different. What is apparent is the significance of the educational process in supporting the development of the paediatric nurse practitioner role. It needs to achieve two purposes; paediatric nurse practitioners graduating from the programme require to be competent to practice and fit for purpose, and they also need to be confident in their own abilities given the realities of working with children.

Another one of the participants from the MPhil/PhD study picked up on the issue of confidence, maintaining that the paediatric nurse practitioners will need to know that they are backed by the organization and by their medical and nursing colleagues. The intimation was that self-confidence will emerge in response to a developing knowledge base, but also through the way their fellow health care providers enable paediatric nurse practitioners to practise. In short, dealing with the responsibility and the risk will be eased by the environment in which they practise. This underlines the significance of other people's views on the role.

Constructions of the paediatric nurse practitioner role

In general terms, the nurse practitioner role has been recognized as a deviant that in time becomes the norm (Ford, 1997). However, the journey between deviance and normality is not necessarily smooth for anyone whose interests are touched by its development. No matter how logical it is that the traditional map of health care provision is redrawn (Doyal and Cameron, 2000) so that the person best able to provide the care delivers it (Walsh, 2000), the nurse practitioner role creates disquiet. There is ample evidence in literature from both the USA and the UK to support this claim. However, it is also apparent that nurse practitioner roles that are planned and clearly understood in terms of what the role will be are less problematic (for example, see Reveley, 1999). That said, Woods (1999) reminds the reader that nurse practitioner roles developing in acute care are contingent on the settings into which they are introduced. Moreover, he found that managers and medical practitioners are instrumental in the process of shaping the nurse practitioner role.

Extrapolating this finding to the local settings, it is quite possible that the paediatric nurse practitioner role will take time to determine its boundaries and its practices and that the paediatric nurse practitioners themselves may be limited in their influence on the final outcome. Leaving this aside for now, given that it has already been acknowledged that the paediatric nurse practitioner initiative is a long-term project, it seems important to reflect on the multiple and competing constructions held in the two settings in respect of the role. It is argued that they are important, if only for their potential to exacerbate tension in the teams. However, before exploring how the role is seen, it is worth stressing that none of the constructs identified in the data is peculiar. The literature is replete with examples of how the nurse practitioner role is viewed. In a perverse way, there is comfort in the fact that the way the paediatric nurse practitioner role is seen in the two local settings is shared across venues in the UK and in the USA.

A few participants saw the paediatric nurse practitioner role as a 'doer of tasks', taking on some of what junior doctors currently do.

More saw the paediatric nurse practitioner role as equivalent to the junior doctor role, effectively taking on all that it comprises. There was an appreciation by a number of participants that children and families would gain from either of these versions of the paediatric nurse practitioner role. It was thought that paediatric nurse practitioners would be better able to undertake the technical components of the role, but would do so in a child- and family-friendly manner. Believing that the paediatric nurse practitioner role would effectively fill the place of the junior doctor, but take to it the skills of children's nursing, enabled a few participants to construct a 'value added' version of the paediatric nurse practitioner role. In this case, the paediatric nurse practitioner was seen as able to contribute more to the care of children and their families than the junior doctor.

On the surface, it appears that the 'value added' construct prizes the skills of children's nursing. However, like the 'doer of tasks' and the 'doctor substitute' constructs, it still seems to align the role to medicine. As a consequence, some participants felt that the paediatric nurse practitioner role does not belong to nursing but to medicine. Therefore, although paediatric nurse practitioners remain nurses, they are not nursing when they practise the role of the paediatric nurse practitioner. Cahill (1995) saw this too, and spoke of nurse practitioner roles medicalizing nursing practice.

Clearly, for Cahill (1995) and for some participants in the study the boundaries of what is and what is not nursing practice are very real. The future of health care provision may look to a far more flexible approach to care delivery, but the traditional map of 'who does what' has yet to be redrawn in everyone's mind. It was apparent in the data that the diagnostic and treatment aspects of the role contributed to the perception that the paediatric nurse practitioner role is medically oriented, but it was also evident that other tasks associated with the paediatric nurse practitioner role aligned it with medicine and not nursing. Examples cited included cannulation, ordering investigations, and doing the paperwork after ward rounds.

There was also a perception that what Doyal and Cameron (2000) identify as 'task drift' on the boundaries of medical and nursing practice was seen to be more of a case of medical staff 'dumping' the work they no longer can or want to do on nurses, as was seen to have happened in the past. Consequently, the paediatric nurse practitioner role to be introduced to the two settings was constructed as medicine in disguise and on the cheap (Cahill, 1995; Edwards, 1995). There were other views in the data.

Less common than the junior doctor replacement or the 'value added' role, but still evident, was the construct of the hybrid. It reflects Barton *et al.*'s (1999) analysis of nurse practitioner roles, which sees the practitioner as a mix of medicine and nursing, effectively creating a new being. One participant saw that the paediatric nurse practitioner operating in this role would be able to build bridges between parents and doctors and between doctors and nurses. They were not alone in perceiving that the paediatric nurse practitioner role could be advantageous to the ward nurses. Another participant believed that paediatric nurse practitioners' prior knowledge of being a ward nurse would enable them to know what ward nurses need and want and to provide it. The idea was that as a result practice would be smoothed for ward nurses and better for children and their families. However, interestingly, this particular participant did not see the paediatric nurse practitioner role as a nursing role.

This raises to the fore the fact that the paediatric nurse practitioner role as planned for the two settings will not look like children's nursing practice as it is currently understood. However, literature from the USA urges caution in pushing the paediatric nurse practitioner role out from the sphere of children's nursing practice because of its appearance. For example, Knaus *et al.* (1997) presented a study that sought to provide insight into nurse practitioners' work in the acute care, non-paediatric setting. It focused on what the nurse practitioners did and gathered data from satisfaction surveys. The nurse practitioner role was described as part of a collaborative practice model developed in a university hospital to assist resident physicians in the co-ordination of patient care. Data were collected on daily work activities and categorized as direct care, indirect care, administration, education or research. Satisfaction surveys gathered data from patients, physicians and nursing staff. Three nurse practitioners were involved in the study; they were each in their first year of practice. Data were collected over a 5-month period.

Knaus *et al.* (1997) reported that 39 per cent of acute care nurse practitioner time was spent delivering direct care, each patient activity averaging 20.7 minutes. Most time was spent in clinic visits and follow-up activities, identified as evaluating laboratory tests or monitoring special tests and procedures. Indirect care accounted for 31 per cent of their time, of which inpatient rounds consumed the largest portion. Knaus *et al.* (1997) noted that, once summed, direct and indirect care account for 70 per cent of the nurse practitioners' time. Of the remainder, 13 per cent was given to administration, 12 per cent to educational activities and 5 per cent to research.

Up to this point, Knaus *et al.'s* (1997) study could be seen as supporting a belief that the nurse practitioner role substitutes for medicine. The data concerning patient care seem to speak of tasks associated with medicine, not nursing. Consequently, the satisfaction data are particularly important, perhaps especially as they relate to patients' views. In brief, patients reported that the nurse practitioners were extremely friendly and concerned for them, were able to make them feel comfortable and were understanding of their concerns. They saw the nurse practitioners' support of them as excellent. In addition, patients thought that the nurse practitioners were extremely helpful in helping them understand medical conditions, tests, procedures and treatments. Of note was the 'timeliness' of the information given to them. Finally, patients reported that nurse practitioners were extremely efficient at procedures and the technical aspects of care.

Knaus *et al.* (1997) also reported on data gathered from attending physicians and residents. They rated nurse practitioners' discharge planning and co-ordination of patient education as very good. Their abilities to develop a plan of care, determine the need for laboratory studies and provide outpatient teaching were rated as good. Nursing staff saw the nurse practitioners' most significant contribution to care as enhanced communication, although it was not clear with whom. Nursing staff also identified the nurse practitioners' ability as a liaison and resource person and patient/family teacher.

The nurse practitioner role featured in this study may have looked like medicine, but it seems that it was delivered through a nursing orientation. Patients were in receipt of the nurse practitioners' technical efficiency, offered through an interpersonal framework that was friendly, made patients feel comfortable and understood their concerns. There is a need to be really careful here and not suggest that doctors are not interpersonally skilled. However, it can be argued that this aspect of medical practice has been devalued in comparison to its core tasks of diagnosis and treatment and, as a result, doctors have concentrated less on building this dimension of their practice.

Perhaps it is that the paediatric nurse practitioner role to be introduced to the two settings will be able to replicate something of what the nurse practitioners in Knaus *et al.'s* (1997) study achieved. Certainly, the patients seemed to value the combination of technical and interpersonal skills. Children and families might too. A second study from the USA suggests this could be the case. Reported by Martin (1999), it focused on the contribution of the nurse practitioner role to children, families and the nursing team in the paediatric critical care setting. The study utilized a convenience sample of parents and staff nurses over a 6-month period, gathering data via questionnaires from both groups. Findings revealed that parents were 'very highly satisfied' with the role of the paediatric critical care nurse practitioner. Comments made were overwhelmingly positive. For example, one parent said:

It was a pleasure and a comfort having someone who really knew my child and was knowledgeable about her illness.

Another parent said:

Overall, I am very appreciative of the wonderful care of all the nurse practitioners, and recommend this programme to other units of the hospital.

All parents indicated that they always felt assured their child received appropriate care from the paediatric critical care nurse practitioner. Staff nurses were equally satisfied with the contribution of the paediatric critical care nurse practitioners, and supported the role. Gaedeke and Blount's (1995) paper adds weight to the claim that in the USA nurse practitioners in paediatric settings are making a positive contribution to the provision of care. They maintain they although paediatric nurse practitioners look as though they are practising medicine, they are more than doctor substitutes because, in addition to taking histories and undertaking physical examination, they bring skills such as education, counselling, accessing resources and promoting health into play. Like some participants in the MPhil/PhD study, they conclude it is a 'value added' role. What makes it unique is its nursing orientation.

Given mounting evidence from the USA, the task force's decision to run with the paediatric nurse practitioner role as planned can be seen as informed. If alternative care models need to be found, then choosing one that has been tested elsewhere seems wise. Yet, despite the fact that literature from the USA supports the paediatric nurse practitioner role, it is clear that in the two settings into which the paediatric nurse practitioner role is to be introduced there is little direct experience of the role. Therefore doctors, nurses and other personnel are always working with what they think the role will be and not what they know it is, and consequently multiple constructions develop, some of which are in direct conflict with one another. The construct of the 'doer of tasks' does not sit easily with the construct of the bridge-building hybrid. Moreover, the role's allegiance to medicine, nursing or neither is a matter of dispute, raising questions about lines of accountability and professional support.

However, uncertainty is a feature of change and perhaps has to be lived with as the role takes shape. As noted, this is a long-term project and there is almost bound to be shift and flux as the role emerges through its students. But, as Woods (1999) contended, key players shape advanced nursing roles, and they are not the nurses themselves. Managers and senior doctors control the process, and the power of nurses to create their own expanded sphere of practice is exposed as being limited (Woods, 1999). However, in effect the paediatric nurse practitioner role envisaged for the two settings has already been decided, and a front-line role demanding the ability to make diagnostic decisions and devise treatment plans is part of the package. Nevertheless, some participants in the MPhil/PhD study indicated that even although this remit is in the

public domain, the role still remain ill-defined. Moreover, it is also recognized by some that expectations of the paediatric nurse practitioners are multiple and competing, reflecting, no doubt, the variety of constructs held by individuals on both sites.

Interestingly, neither the expectations held of the paediatric nurse practitioners nor the various constructs of the role can be attributed to particular professional groups. Quite simply, individuals see this role very differently, and their professional background does not dictate the way they see it. In amongst all this variety and the potential that seems inherent in the role, one wonders where children's nursing will feature in the role still to take shape? Perhaps it is just the foundation for paediatric nurse practitioner practice. In the two local settings, students accepted on to the course have to be on either Parts 8 or 15 of the Professional Register, and they have to be experienced. However, the front-line role envisaged for them does not prescribe how this background will be used and, as acknowledged earlier, there is doubt in some people's minds that it will be drawn on at all.

Of course, if children's nursing is not integral to paediatric nurse practitioner practice it begs the question, why pursue a paediatric nurse practitioner option? A physician's assistant was another possibility, as is employed in paediatric settings in the USA. Presumably, the task force perceived that children's nurses had something to offer to the role, beyond the fact of their professional registration. However, exactly which aspects of children's nursing practice were valued as part of the paediatric nurse practitioner role was not stated. Even so, it must have been imagined that children's nurses could contribute to the service and benefit children and families. This said, quite how children and families will see the role is a matter of debate amongst participants. Parents at one site may have petitioned to keep their local inpatient service, but the task force has pursued the paediatric nurse practitioner option without engaging in consultation with either children or families. Presumably it was confident that the paediatric nurse practitioner role would be well received, yet children's and families' acceptance or rejection of the role can determine its fate. This then leads to the question as to what matters to children and families when they access health services? On the basis of what matters, the role might take shape whilst still working towards providing the 'front-line' activities embracing the skills of diagnostic reasoning and clinical decision making. In order better to understand the consumer perspective, attention is first drawn to three studies, those by Kai (1996), Kristensson-Hallstrom and Elander (1997) and Price (1993). Each in different ways affords insight into what is important for service users.

Kai (1996)

Kai's (1996) study was situated in primary care and gathered data from 95 parents of pre-school children, focusing on what worries them when their child is acutely ill. The setting was a disadvantaged inner city community area in the UK. Interviews were used to gather the data. The study found that the parents' priority, what mattered to them, was to monitor and maintain control of symptoms in order to minimize the child's discomfort and reduce the risk of harm and fear of death. It was this that made them seek professional help, even although they felt guilty about bothering people and ignorant in the face of professional knowledge. What mattered was getting help for their child, for whom they acknowledged an acute sense of responsibility; that was their focus of interest – their child. Talk of relationships with professionals did not feature in the report of the study. This said, Kai (1996) identified the potential for communication breakdown between parents and professionals because the knowledge base employed by the two groups quite often differs, with the result that professionals may not appreciate the level and source of parental concern. For example, parents in the study attributed risk to certain symptoms in a way that was not necessarily logical but was nevertheless very real to them. Therefore, the child with a fever but without an accompanying symptom was a source of considerable worry, provoking acute anxiety. Yet, to the professional, the same child may be of minimal concern. Kai (1996) concludes by urging professionals to understand parental perspectives in order to promote more effective communication. This is hard to argue with,

but the potential limitations of the study in terms of its sampling need to be recognized and allowed for in any generalization to health care provision.

Kristensson-Hallstrom and Elander, 1997

The second study is limited in its utility for similar reasons, but still has the ability to enable better understanding to develop in respect of what matters to the parents of hospitalized children. Conducted in Sweden, it involved interviewing the parents of 20 boys aged 2–14 years admitted for surgery. It found that what was most important to the parents was to find security at the hospital. Parents manifested one of three strategies in order to achieve this outcome: the first involved relinquishing the care of their child to nursing staff; the second required them to be able to gain a measure of control over their child's care; and the third relied on knowing their child best. Interestingly, the researchers found that the strategy adopted to feel secure corresponded with the way parents experienced the hospitalization. Kristensson-Hallstrom and Elander (1997) conclude by citing Darbyshire (1994):

Nurses need a deeper understanding of the nature of parents' experiences and how these relate to their own nursing practices.

They continue, noting that although children's nurses wish to work with families, the parental role is poorly defined in hospital and therefore gives rise to stress for the families and conflict with the staff. Developing services for children and families, they say, must account for individual differences in need, within and across family groups, a conclusion that leads into the third study focused on parental perceptions of quality.

Price, 1993

Price's (1993) research was small and described as qualitative. From an identified sample of six parents, three mothers and one father agreed to be interviewed. The time since their children had been in hospital ranged from 16 months to 7 years. The data suggest that what parents experience as quality nursing care involves a four-stage process:

1. Manoeuvring
2. The process of knowing
3. Positive relationships
4. Quality nursing care.

Price's (1993) elaborations of each of these four phases offers insight not only into parental perceptions of quality, but also into their views of what is important and what they are prepared to do to achieve a particular goal, namely the development of a positive relationship with the nurse. So, for example, manoeuvring was identified as a strategy designed to draw nurses to the child's bedside so they could get to know each other. To achieve this, parents would 'help' the nurses and 'be nice' to them. Price (1993) also identified nurse behaviours likely to interfere with a family's manoeuvring strategy; these were described as 'nurse technical' and 'nurse repelling'. Both were seen to represent a non-child or non-parent focused approach to care. The first perceived the nurse to be overly concerned with the technical components of care and not the child or family, and the second saw the nurse as not wishing to engage with the family.

What emerges from Price's (1993) study overall is the significance of a positive relationship between the nurse and the family. It was perceived to benefit both the child and the parents, and made a difference to the hospital stay. It was not that other components of the role of the nurse, described primarily as the technical aspects of care, were unimportant, it was simply that a positive relationship was viewed as a necessary foundation for quality health care provision. Achieving the goal required contact with the nurse, and was something that parents were prepared to engineer.

It is possible to interpret these findings in different ways. Certainly the fact that the hospitalization event was not recent, and for one parent occurred 7 years previously, is probably significant. Time and subsequent experience can alter perceptions of events and reconfigure the relative importance of what matters. Even so, in their recall of the hospitalization event with their child their need for a positive relationship with the nurse featured, so too did their memories of nurses who did not offer quality care.

What matters?

Taken together, these three studies illuminate something of what matters to parents, if not to children themselves. Clearly they may have fears and concerns, but might prefer not to bother people and can feel ignorant in the face of professional knowledge (Kai, 1996). They may need to feel secure, but how they achieve this end could require the use of particular strategies that serve to illustrate the individuality of parents and their needs (Kristensson-Hallstrom and Elander, 1997). They may value nurses who spend time with them getting to know the child, and might be able to identify nurses who are oriented to technical tasks and away from families (Price, 1993).

In their quest to enable parents to get involved and participate in their child's care, in their need to provide family-centred care and form partnerships, children's nurses could learn from what seems to matter to parents in these three studies. However, the role of the paediatric nurse practitioner, planned for introduction to the two local settings, might also be informed by what seems to matter to parents. As was noted at the beginning of the chapter, change has to be in the parents' interests and those of their child. If not, its implementation should be questioned. With this in mind, 13 interviews were carried out in May 2000. The sample was convenient, and drew 12 mothers and two children into the study over a 4-day period to try to understand what is important to them and whether they would have been happy to see a paediatric nurse practitioner when they first came into hospital.

They spoke of many things; however, without doubt the parents valued nurses who talked to them, kept them up to date, showed them where things were and explained what they needed to do. They valued contact with them, and appreciated it when nurses showed interest in their children and worked to build a relationship with them. The interpersonal skills of the children's nurse were important to the mothers. They were also mentioned by one of the children interviewed. Mothers also spoke about wanting a diagnosis as soon as possible, getting treatment started and getting back home. They wanted the best care for their children.

Asked how they would feel about their

children seeing a paediatric nurse practitioner rather than a doctor on admission, thoughts varied. For some parents it did not matter; in fact one mother could see advantages:

It would have been fine with me, because really when we first came in we just wanted to see one person that can ask you all the questions, assess you and give you the information that you need to know all at once, instead of dealing with maybe three or four people at a time.

Another mother felt that seeing a paediatric nurse practitioner would be better:

Personally, I would feel better actually. Sometimes you feel like you can't talk to doctors. You can talk to the nurse; she's not going to be offhand. Sometimes, doctors, I'm not saying they're tired or anything, but they sort of, you feel like you're imposing on them.

However, not everyone was agreed on this. One mother said that she would not be happy for her child to be seen by a paediatric nurse practitioner:

... in my head there's a big difference between the doctor and the nurse, between the two. And you want the better qualified person to be assessing them. ... I have to have complete faith in the doctor ... if the nurse had said that it wouldn't be the same.

Interestingly, this mother's son, after thinking about it, decided that his acceptance of the paediatric nurse practitioner would depend on the individual:

... So I wouldn't say, 'right, you're just a nurse, go away, come here, doctor'. If I thought the nurse was alright, yeah, I'd have the nurse.

For another mother, whether she would be happy or not with seeing a paediatric nurse practitioner would depend upon the reason for seeking health care. However, the data suggest that it would be a mistake to assume that the sicker the child was perceived to be, the less happy the parents would be for their child to see a nurse. The data indicated that mothers seek health care for their child when there is a gap between what they can offer and what the child needs. It depends on whether or not the mother thinks the paediatric nurse practitioner can fill the gap. If she thinks the nurse practitioner can, she might accept or even welcome seeing one.

It is important to stress that the sample was convenient and none of the parents or children had actually experienced the care of one of the paediatric nurse practitioner students. Nevertheless, the data are rich and justice cannot be done to them here. What is of note is that what they said did not contradict the findings of the three studies featured earlier. Perhaps even more important is that the interview data suggest that if the two settings are determined to develop their services through the paediatric nurse practitioner role, then there is an opportunity to do so. Parents want the interpersonal component of care that they associate with nurses, but they also want explanations, a diagnosis, reassurance, and to get back home. The enhanced knowledge base of the paediatric nurse practitioner combined with their skills of working with children and families may enable the role to do more than fill the gap being exposed by changes in medical cover. Therefore, it could be a role worth its investment.

However, it does provoke tension and will likely do so as it continues to take shape over time. Analysis of the interview data gathered from the paediatric nurse practitioner students and the health care providers hints at the possibility that for some participants the role would be easier to come to terms with if it were pushed beyond the margins of what is deemed to be nursing practice and consigned to the edge of medicine. This might be less threatening to nurses and more capable of being controlled by doctors. Yet not all nurses seemed threatened by it, and not all doctors wished to control it. Indeed, one medical practitioner said:

It's not just a case of 'we haven't got doctors, we'll have nurse practitioners and that will solve the problem in 3 years' time'. If that's how they are thinking, it will just spiral down to nothingness really.

For this individual, the paediatric nurse practitioner role had to be more than a replacement doctor. Only then could it impact on the service for the well-being of consumers and providers. The belief was that it offered the potential to make a positive contribution to health care provision. Furthermore, it was seen by this participant to be a role that advanced nursing practice. This is an important conclusion because if the role is claimed by children's nursing, then it offers a route for continuing professional development in a field of practice that Glasper (1995), among others, believes struggles in its search for career advancement. Although this should not be the reason for the development of the paediatric nurse practitioner role, it is a positive outcome.

However, in order that the paediatric nurse practitioner role can be an advancement of children's nursing practice, it has to be seen as something that grows around and through what it is that children's nurses already offer to health care provision. It cannot be that the role is simply convenient as a base on which to build something else; that would not value children's nursing as a sphere of practice. Paradoxically, it is likely that constructing the paediatric nurse practitioner role as an advancement of children's nursing will threaten at least a few children's nurses. Any attempt to present the paediatric nurse practitioner role as a new and improved version of children's nursing could well alienate individuals who choose not to pursue the route. The needs of the nurses 'left behind', as one participant put it, cannot afford to be ignored. Neither can the paediatric nurse practitioners' impact on doctors be neglected. Consideration of the impact of the role on medical colleagues is now offered in brief. The lens employed is intentionally narrow, focusing on the practice setting and the need for student paediatric nurse practitioners to learn and develop their skills. Crumbie offers more depth to other educational issues in Chapter 9.

Educating the paediatric nurse practitioner in the clinical setting: lessons from experience

Just as was the case in the USA, until such time as the paediatric nurse practitioner movement has developed its own educators who can support student paediatric nurse practitioners in the clinical setting, it is necessary to draw on the services of senior medical staff. However, these medical facilitators are asked to fit the role round their existing clinical responsibilities and the requirement that they support junior doctors and more recently staff grades. It is an onerous task that demands time and commitment. It also requires flexibility on behalf of the consultant paediatricians. They are confronted with a nursing orientation to the process of practice-based education that brings with it

learning contracts, competence profiles and tripartite arrangements with nurse educationalists to monitor students' progress. It is all a little foreign, and its strangeness for medical colleagues was not really fully appreciated until quite recently. Yet, as Hunter and Walsh (1999) maintain, it is vital that both the academic and the practice-based components of nurse practitioner courses are orchestrated by nursing. Only then can the role be sure to advance through a nursing framework that values what nursing is and can be (Hopkins, 1996).

It has been necessary and instructive to work with medical colleagues in what will be a temporary arrangement. In time, paediatric nurse practitioners will support their own students. There is tension in the process and a need to keep a firm grip on what the role is, even if it is seen in another way. Achieving this has been enabled by a competence profile that draws on competence statements devised in the USA to set the standards for paediatric nurse practitioner practice. These statements offer a benchmark and, moreover, ensure that the nursing element of the role does not get lost in the development of skills previously associated with medical practice.

If the early days of the development of the paediatric nurse practitioner role have demanded the creation of partnerships between consultant paediatricians and nurse educationalists, they have also required consideration of the learning needs of junior doctors. In effect, when student paediatric nurse practitioners are on their practice day they are in competition with the junior doctors for learning experiences. More and more emphasis is being placed on the need for junior doctors' learning to be targeted on what they need to know, and not on being a service provider. This brings the student paediatric nurse practitioner and the junior doctor into the same space, and there are only so many children to learn with. Quite possibly this highlights one of the major differences between the development of nurse practitioner roles in GP practices in primary care settings and those emerging in the hospital environment. It would be an unusual day for there to be just a few appointments booked in to see the general practitioner. By contrast, children's wards can be exceedingly quiet or extremely busy. Neither situation makes for well-organized learning under supervision. The learning environment available to nurse practitioner students in primary and acute care seems different; both have to be worked with to enable competence to develop and confidence to grow. Achieving this goal for the paediatric nurse practitioner students demands lateral thinking in terms of whom they can learn with and where they might access experience. Rather than being a disadvantage, getting the students to move out of the children's ward can be seen as beneficial. It gets the role known, facilitates networking and affords the paediatric nurse practitioners a breadth of vision that extends beyond the domain of the children's ward.

Conclusion

There are many other aspects of the paediatric nurse practitioner role planned for the two settings that could be examined. However, perhaps the issues most important to the journey so far have been explored. At the time of writing the role is just 8 months old, developing through its students who are pioneering its place in two small district general hospitals. There is uncertainty and tension, but both are inevitable. Change does that. Nothing remains the same. Reflection suggests that if it can be argued that this is a role with the potential to benefit children and families, then it must be pursued. However, its development should not damage other people or roles. Neither should its growth demean the field of practice from which it originates and through which, it is argued, it should still develop. The paediatric nurse practitioner role is not an abandonment of children's nursing. Nevertheless, it can challenge those who choose not to pursue its path. This said, children's nursing cannot afford to be static in this world that proposes revolution. Paediatric nurse practitioners and children's nurses could do worse than work together to find out what it is that really matters to children and families, and devise ways of working together to offer what is sought. They are not adversaries, but partners. Service managers and nurse educationalists must collaborate to promote the relationship that promises much, but could be stumbled by fear of the unknown. It is a brave new world, and it is better to travel together than alone. Who knows, we may surprise ourselves and find we can walk with our medical colleagues in pursuit of the same purpose.

Commentary by an American paediatric nurse practitioner lecturer

The following commentary is provided by Janet A. Deatrick, a paediatric nurse practitioner lecturer at the University of Pennsylvania.

The questions raised by Fiona Smart are similar to my own persistent questions during the past 10 years at the University of Pennsylvania. The faculty of the paediatric acute/chronic care and paediatric critical care advanced practice nursing programmes pushed the boundaries of education, practice and regulation in 1992 to begin new paediatric advanced practice programmes. These programmes prepare nurses to practise with children who have serious acute and chronic conditions in advanced practice roles with skills consolidated from both nurse practitioners and clinical nurse specialists. In 1997, a concentration was added to the acute/chronic care programme in paediatric oncology. During the past year, the neonatal nurse practitioner programme was added to this paediatric cluster. The paediatric primary care programme remains housed with the primary care programme.

The anticipated and unanticipated sources of resistance and strain were remarkable during the initial development and implementation of the new programme. However, with more than 300 graduates currently in practice with populations of vulnerable children and their families, the sheer volume of nursing power cannot be denied.

Is every graduate practising from a nursing model? Are their views about care consistent with the priorities perceived by the children and families? Do they meet resistance from other nurses, physicians, and administrators?

The obvious answer to these questions could be discouraging to everyone involved in paediatric practice and education. However, lest we become too discouraged, I believe that there is much reason for hope not only in the present reality but also in the future potential of the paediatric nurse practitioner role across settings.

Since I have the benefit of our history over the past 10 years, I can offer a little wisdom that may be helpful to all those involved in the introduction of the paediatric nurse practitioner role into the children's wards of the district general hospitals discussed above:

1. Concentrate educational experiences on the focus of care rather than the setting of care. For instance, many children with serious illnesses are now able to be maintained in the home and the community rather than in the hospital. Therefore, where these paediatric nurse practitioners deliver the care is a moot point. Rather, the constellation of care concerns of a particular population are of utmost concern. As Fiona Smart states above, we need first to be concerned with the needs and priorities of the patients and their families. Where that care is delivered at a particular point in time will then help us determine the necessary resources and planning.

2. Education of the paediatric nurse practitioner needs to include how that advanced practice nurse relates to other nurses in terms of teaching, leadership, consultation and research. These are the nurse's value added components of practice. I believe that this strategy is critical to the eventual success of the role for influencing children's health care. If the paediatric nurse practitioner practises only on a one-to-one basis with particular children and families, their spheres of possible influence will not be realized beyond a medical model. Ways to incorporate staff or ward nurses into the education of a paediatric nurse practitioner include joint projects, nursing rounds, ward leadership projects, and consultations that are planned and evaluated and given the same priority as histories, physical examinations and clinical decision making. While students are most anxious to learn these technical skills, they are only part of the paediatric nurse practitioner role.

3. Education of the paediatric nurse practitioner needs to include content and experiences related to child and family development. The traditional role of the primary care paediatric nurse practitioner has always had its foundation in anticipatory guidance related to the developing child and family. This cannot be lost because the child is in the hospital or because the child is ill. Again, the sphere of our influence will be considerably lessened and children's health care will be negatively affected.

References

Annandale E. and Clark, J. (1996). What is gender? Feminist theory and the sociology of human reproduction. *Sociol. Health Illness*, **18(1)**, 17–44.

Barton, T. D., Thorn, R., Hoptroff, D. *et al.* (1999). The nurse practitioner; redefining occupational boundaries? *Int. J. Nursing Studies*, **36**, 57–63.

Brush, B. L. and Capezuti, E. A. (1996). Revisiting 'a nurse for all settings': the nurse practitioner movement 1965–1995. *J. Am. Acad. NPs*, **8(1)**, 5–10.

Cahill, H. (1995). Role definition; nurse practitioners and clinical assistants? *Br. J. Nursing*, **5(22)**, 1382–5.

Calkin, J. D. (1984). A model for advanced nursing practice. *J. Nursing Admin.*, **Jan**, 24–30.

Callaghan, N., Evans, J., Caldwell, C. *et al.* (1997). Reflections on nurse-led day cases. *Paed. Nursing*, **9(8)**, 14–17.

Davies, C. (2000). Vive la différence; that's what will make collaboration work. *Nursing Times*, **96(15)**, 27.

Dearmun, A. and Gordon, K. (1999). The nurse practitioner in children's ambulatory care. *Paed. Nursing*, **11(1)**, 18–21.

Department of Health (2000). *The National Health Service Plan: A Plan for Improvement, a Plan for Reform*. Stationery Office.

Dickson, N. (1996). Debate: are nurse practitioners merely substitute doctors? *Prof. Nurse*, **11(5)**, 325–8.

Doyal, L. and Cameron, A. (2000). Reshaping the NHS workforce. *Br. Med. J.*, **320**, 1023–4.

Edwards, K. (1995). What are nurses' views of expanding practice? *Nursing Standard*, **9(41)**, 38–40.

Ford, L. C. (1997). A deviant comes of age. *Heart Lung*, **26(2)**, 87–91.

Gaedeke, M. K. and Blount, K. (1995). Advanced practice nursing in pediatric acute care. *Crit. Care Nursing Clin. North Am.*, **7(1)**, 61–9.

Glasper, E. A. (1995). Prescribing children's nursing in a climate of genericism. *Br. J. Nursing*, **4(1)**, 24–5.

Hopkins, S. (1996). Junior doctors' hours and the expanding role of the nurse. *Nursing Times*, **92(14)**, 35–6.

Hughes, E. (1998). In: *Classic Texts in Health Care* (L. Mackay and K. Soothill, eds). Butterworth-Heinemann.

Hunter, P. and Walsh, M. (1999). The Importance of education. *Nursing Standard/J. RCN NP Assoc.*, **13(46)**, 49–50.

Hutton, W. (2000). *New Life for Health: The Commission on the NHS*. Vintage.

Kai, J. (1996). What warns parents when their pre-school children are acutely ill and why; a qualitative study. *Br. Med. J.*, **313**, 983–6.

Knaus, V. L., Felten, S., Burton, S. *et al.* (1997). The use of nurse practitioners in the acute care setting. *J. Nursing Admin.*, **27(2)**, 20–27.

Kobryn, M. and Pearce, S. (1991). The paediatric nurse practitioner. *Paed. Nursing*, **June**, Vol 3, Issue 5, 11–14.

Kristensson-Hallstrom, I. and Elander, G. (1997). Parents' experience of hospitalization: different strategies for feeling secure. *Ped. Nursing*, **23(4)**, 361–7.

Martin, S. A. (1999). The pediatric critical care nurse practitioner; evolution and impact. *Ped. Nursing*, **25(5)**, 505–10.

Miller, S. K. (1998). Refining the acute in acute care nurse practitioners. *Clin. Excellence NPs*, **2(1)**, 52–5.

Price, P. J. (1993). Parents' perceptions of the meaning of quality nursing care. *Adv. Nursing Sci.*, **16(1)**, 33–41.

Reveley, S. (1999). Introducing the nurse practitioner into general medical practice: theoretical and operational perspectives on the role. Unpublished PhD thesis, University of Lancaster.

Walsh, M. (2000). *Nursing Frontiers: Accountability and the Boundaries of Care*. Butterworth-Heinemann.

Woods, L. P. (1999). The contingent nature of advanced nursing practice. *J. Adv. Nursing*, **30(1)**, 121–8.

8

THE PRIMARY/SECONDARY CARE INTERFACE: MINOR INJURIES, ACCIDENT AND EMERGENCY AND OTHER SERVICES

Mike Walsh

Though leaves are many, the root is one
From *The Coming of Wisdom with Time*,
by W. B. Yeats (1910)

Introduction

There are many different ways that the nurse practitioner can impact upon improving hospital care, but all share the common root of increased autonomy of practice. Nowhere is this better illustrated than in the treatment of patients in the accident and emergency department or the minor injuries unit. The nurse practitioner role first made a significant impact on the hospital sector in these areas. This chapter will not only discuss the role within these familiar settings, but will also explore how nurse practitioners can base themselves in these areas but offer new and innovative services to the public. This discussion will underline Yeats's observation quoted above, for there are indeed many nurse practitioner roles but all are underpinned by the same common principles.

It is well recognized that accident and emergency departments have become serious pressure points within the National Health Service, and are the first parts of the service to bear the brunt of any major problems such as the annual 'winter pressures' crisis. Medical staffing remains problematic, and the stress and pressure on nursing staff inevitably takes its toll. Approximately one-third of the population will visit an accident and emergency department every year. Lengthy waits for treatment of 4–6 hours are commonplace, whilst every winter we have the disgraceful situation of sick patients spending 24 hours or more on trolleys in accident and emergency departments waiting for beds. During 2000, the government recognized the importance of improving accident and emergency services as part of its plans to modernize the NHS and has

pledged major funding towards rebuilding run-down accident and emergency departments. The National Health Service Plan, published in July 2000, states that there will be an end to lengthy waits, promising that by 2004 nobody should wait for longer than 4 hours in an accident and emergency department (Donnelly *et al.*, 2000).

Initiatives and promises such as these are welcome. However, new ways of working and delivering services, such as that offered by the nurse practitioner, are necessary if we are to meet the government's objectives. This may be by developing a new role within conventional services or by utilizing the special environment of the minor injuries unit/accident and emergency department as a base to offer a new range of services. A unique feature of accident and emergency is that it is on the interface of primary and secondary care and offers a convenient drop-in facility. This of course helps to explain why the service becomes so overloaded. However, this problem can be turned to our advantage as health care providers, as we shall see later in this chapter.

The current situation

Two distinct patterns of service provision can be discerned (Walsh, 2000). First, the large accident and emergency department may employ nurses to provide a fast-track service for patients with minor injuries and ailments, thereby bypassing the doctor. This frees up scarce medical time and allows doctors to concentrate on treating those patients with more serious conditions. Effective triage should ensure that those patients who are appropriate for independent nursing management treatment are seen by the nurse. This model has developed extensively in emergency departments in the USA, where rigorous research shows that nurse practitioners can not only speed up treatment of minor injuries but also treat a similar range of patients to doctors within a similar time scale, and with equally good outcomes (Blunt, 1998). Buchanan and Powers (1997) report that their graduate emergency nurse practitioners see 21 per cent of patients who attend the emergency department, consistently achieving very high internal audit scores. The most telling statistic is perhaps that in the 18 years they have operated a fast-track emergency nurse practitioner service, not a single lawsuit has been filed against an emergency nurse practitioner (Buchanan and Powers, 1997).

The second scenario, which has developed in the UK, is the provision of nurse-led services in minor injuries units. In some instances these are former accident and emergency departments that have been closed down as medical staffing has been withdrawn and services centralized on a larger accident and emergency department. Alternatively, nurse-led services are based in community hospitals where nurses have effectively been providing the service informally for many years, backed up by varying degrees of general practitioner cover.

The UK literature describing these services uses a variety of terms such as 'nurse practitioner', 'nurse-led' and, increasingly, 'emergency nurse practitioner'. This reflects the uncertainty in the UK over the use of the term nurse practitioner and its definition. In the USA, the term emergency nurse practitioner is widespread and refers to a nurse who has undertaken a formal university educational programme, usually at Masters level. A typical course is offered in Texas and described by Cole (1998). It consists of 21 months of full-time study at Masters level, and over 800 hours of supervised clinical practice. The course philosophy is to equip the nurse to manage, as the first point of contact, a patient presenting with any condition from a minor injury to a serious emergency. The title 'emergency nurse practitioner' is therefore an accurate description of the work the nurse undertakes.

Problems arise, however, when UK nurses adopt the emergency nurse practitioner title. In most cases they have little formal educational preparation and are only treating minor injuries, working within strict protocols and guidelines. The majority of nurses using the title emergency nurse practitioner in this country are not managing patients who are emergencies, and do not possess a formal nurse practitioner educational qualification. The title is therefore inappropriate in many instances. This issue of title and educational preparation for the role is a continuing problem running throughout both the literature and practice of nursing in the accident and emergency environment in the UK. The points made above should be borne in mind whilst reading the rest of this chapter, as the term emergency nurse practitioner will occur frequently, reflecting its commonplace usage in the UK literature.

An illuminating picture of the emergency nurse practitioner fast-track approach has been painted by Tye *et al.* (1998) in their national survey, actually carried out in 1996. This postal survey of all 293 major accident and emergency departments in the UK produced an excellent response rate of 94 per cent, and showed that 36 per cent of departments had a formal emergency nurse practitioner fast-track service of some kind, while a further 33 per cent stated an intention to introduce such a scheme. Marked geographical variations were found, with the highest level of provision being in the London area (just over 50 per cent) and the lowest in Scotland (14 per cent). A serious matter for concern, however, was that of those departments who stated they had a fast-track emergency nurse practitioner service, only 27 per cent stated that the staff involved were dedicated to such a service. In other words, staff in 73 per cent of units had to combine traditional nursing duties with their emergency nurse practitioner role.

This has serious implications for the quality of the service provided. The nurse practitioner role is fundamentally different from that of the registered nurse, and requires different skills. It is therefore unreasonable to expect a nurse continually to switch between the two. Nurse practitioner skills need to be practised and consolidated; experience has to built up and reflected upon for further learning to occur. Neither of these processes can occur if the nurse is prevented from working consistently in the nurse practitioner role. If a nurse has developed extensive nurse practitioner skills, especially if a formal degree-level education has been undertaken, these will be wasted if he or she is expected to operate in a traditional registered nurse role. The nurse is also likely to find this very frustrating and demoralizing.

This point is developed further by Robinson and Inyang (1999), who have shown that the nurse practitioner can make a major contribution to accident and emergency services. Robinson and Inyang (1999) argue that nurse practitioner posts should be seen as a new resource and supported by appropriate funding in addition to the existing nursing establishment. Failure to do this will see the nurse practitioner diverted to routine nursing work, ironically when the department is busiest and the benefit of the nurse practitioner is potentially greatest. The beneficial impact of the nurse practitioner will therefore be lost unless the post is established as a full-time position, separate from the regular nurse staffing roster.

The survey by Tye *et al.* (1998) is very valuable, as it reveals the unsatisfactory state of educational preparation that exists for emergency nurse practitioners. It shows an extremely wide range of education for the role, ranging from none at all to Honours level degree education. Sixty per cent of departments report they only provide a short, in-house training course, typically of 1 to 2 weeks' duration. We can only agree with Tye *et al.* (1998) when they point out that, in view of the high levels of autonomy that the emergency nurse practitioner may be granted, this is inadequate. The survey also revealed extensive use of protocols, which in many cases were so restrictive that the emergency nurse practitioner had, in practice, very little autonomy. This is a logical consequence of inadequate educational preparation for the role, and is demonstrated by statistics such as only 36 per cent of departments reporting allowing their emergency nurse practitioners to interpret X-rays, although almost all those who had emergency nurse practitioners allowed them to order radiographs. Barely half the departments allowed their emergency nurse practitioners to use group protocols to supply and administer a limited range of prescription-only medicines, and only 68 per cent allowed emergency nurse practitioners to supply 'over the counter' medication under protocol. Practice is therefore being severely restricted in many cases, especially when compared with the scope of practice enjoyed by emergency nurse practitioners in the USA.

These kind of data reveal a serious flaw with emergency nurse practitioner provision in the UK at present. Inadequate educational preparation leads to a restrictive scope of practice, which in turn leads in many cases to the nurse being placed in the unsatisfactory position of having to double up as an emergency nurse practitioner and a general nurse. If the range of patients and conditions that can be seen is too limited, it is not possible to justify full-time emergency nurse practitioner posts and so the nurse has to carry on with regular nursing work, preventing achievement of his or her full potential as an emergency nurse practitioner.

Evaluation of nurse-led (emergency nurse practitioner) services in the UK

Although nurse-led services have been widely introduced in minor injuries units and accident and emergency departments, evaluation of these services has been patchy, with few rigorous studies carried out. A summary of recent reports by Walsh (2000) shows that both types of service have been written up in the journals. These reports may be summarized as follows:

- Little audit data on nurse practitioner performance is available, although that which is presented is favourable
- There are no data on cost effectiveness
- There is a lack of formalized education and heavy reliance upon protocols
- Services concentrate upon minor injuries only
- Problems were frequently encountered with other staff groups resisting setting up the service.
- Patient satisfaction where it has been measured is high, and there is no doubt the services are meeting a real need.
- Few formal and therefore rigorous evaluations have been undertaken.

In view of the last point, this section will concentrate on the limited number of studies where rigorous evaluations have been carried out, starting with perhaps the most rigorous, conducted by Sakr *et al.* (1999) in Sheffield. This study concentrated on emergency nurse practitioners providing a fast-track service to patients with minor injuries within a large accident and emergency department. A large sample of 1453 patients were allocated at random to either a nurse practitioner ($n = 704$) or a junior doctor ($n = 749$) for assessment and treatment. Each patient was then seen by a research registrar, who carried out an independent assessment. The registrar's findings were then compared with the initial assessment, which was presented in a masked form so that the person comparing the two did not know whether the patient had seen a nurse or a doctor. This has the value of being a prospective study with real patients rather than a retrospective study based on case notes, coupled with the further strength of random allocation from a large sample. The nurse practitioners in this study had a minimum of 4 years' experience in accident and emergency and, crucially, were undertaking or had completed a formal educational programme, the ENB A33 course, Developing Autonomous Practice.

The results showed that clinically important errors occurred in 9.2 per cent of the patients seen by the emergency nurse practitioner and 10.7 per cent of those seen by the junior doctor. This difference is not statistically significant. A smaller observational study observed the length of time that was required for a consultation (46 nurse practitioner patients and 48 junior doctor patients). The average nurse practitioner consultation was 10.89 minutes compared to 9.02 minutes for a doctor (Sakr *et al.*, 1999).

There are several important conclusions from these data, the main one of which is that properly trained nurse practitioners in accident and emergency are as competent as doctors in the assessment and management of minor injuries. This statement covers examination, radiography requests and interpretation, treatment and planned follow-up of patients. The second conclusion is that junior doctors make significant mistakes in 10 per cent of the minor injuries cases they see in accident and emergency. This should be borne in mind in future studies of the emergency nurse practitioner where they are compared to junior doctors, as a 10 per cent error rate would appear to be no worse than would be expected from junior medical staff. Furthermore, judgements regarding treatment to be used as a benchmark to assess the emergency nurse

practitioner performance should not be made by senior house officers, but by senior medical staff.

Sakr *et al.* (1999) acknowledge that over time the error rate of junior doctors would decrease with increased experience; however, in reality the rotation of junior medical staff ensures they are never in accident and emergency for more than 6 months. That argument is therefore of little value. It could also be argued that the error rate of emergency nurse practitioners would also decrease over time with more experience. These findings are consistent with the work of Meek *et al.* (1998) and Barr *et al.* (2000). The former study reported that nurse practitioners were as good as experienced senior house officers in interpreting X-rays, and actually better than inexperienced senior house officers. A key observation by Meek *et al.* (1998) was that better education would probably improve the performance of all staff, nursing and medical, in ordering and interpreting radiographs.

The adoption of the Ottawa Ankle Rules (OAR) by nurse practitioners (Walsh *et al.*, 1999) has greatly aided their performance in the field of radiography requests for ankle injuries. This is demonstrated by Allerton and Justham (2000a), who report on a series of 354 consecutive patients attending accident and emergency departments with ankle injuries. Nurse practitioners saw 187 patients and applied the OAR in all cases, resulting in 61.5 per cent being sent for X-ray. Medical staff saw 168 patients and requested X-rays in 80.4 per cent of cases, a highly significant difference. In the nurse practitioner group 29.6 per cent of patients had a fracture, compared to 22.8 per cent of those requested by medical staff. These findings are consistent with the work of Salt and Clancy (1997) and Mann *et al.* (1998), who have both shown that nurse practitioners can apply the OAR to reduce substantially the number of patients being sent for unnecessary X-rays. Mann *et al.* (1998) did report, however, that five fractures were missed out of a group of 1365 patients. This error rate of 0.4 per cent should be compared with the rates cited above in the study by Sakr *et al.* (1999). Nurse practitioners applying OAR therefore result in a significant reduction in the number of radiographs being ordered, and hence cost and time savings.

Sakr *et al.* (1999) also found that the nurse practitioner took 1.5 minutes longer than the junior doctor to see patients. This difference, while statistically significant ($p < 0.05$), is of little operational significance and reflects the different nature of the nurse practitioner consultation. It refutes suggestions that nurse practitioners take far longer than doctors to see patients, but also confirms the view that nurse practitioners are not a cheap substitute for medical staff either. When the average salary per hour for the nurses in this study (F grade) was compared with the senior house officers, the medical service worked out slightly cheaper. However, the advantages to the department and to the patient of operating a nurse-led fast-track service were so great that this was felt to be a small price to pay.

The impact of the nurse practitioner in speeding up treatment has been reported by Barr *et al.* (2000). In their accident and emergency department they found the mean waiting time to see the nurse practitioner was 22 minutes, compared with 86 minutes to see a doctor. A further example of the advantages to be derived from a nurse practitioner fast-track service has been reported by Allerton and Justham (2000b). They showed that nurse practitioners applying the OAR directly at triage reduced transit times in the accident and emergency department by an average of 20–25 minutes. The study does not comment on the educational preparation of the nurse practitioners involved, but rather tellingly notes that two nurse practitioners did not use the OAR because they felt uncomfortable in doing so and did not wish to extend their scope of practice. Comments such as these are not really consistent with nurse practitioner status, and raise the possibility of experienced nurses being pushed into roles they are not educationally equipped for.

The different nature of the emergency nurse practitioner–patient consultation has been highlighted by Dolan (2000), who has piloted tools that may be used to investigate this further. Such work would be very welcome, for if the emergency nurse practitioner is not be viewed as a direct substitute for a doctor, it is necessary to demonstrate how the emergency nurse practitioner consultation is intrinsically different.

Nurse-led minor injuries unit services have been carefully evaluated at a community hospital in Horsham, West Sussex (Mabrook and Dale, 1998), and on the site of a former accident and emergency unit in Edinburgh (Heaney and Paxton, 1997). Both projects were characterized by significant opposition from within the NHS (particularly the medical profession in Edinburgh) when they were established, as well as unease amongst the general public. The need for a substantial public awareness campaign that also involves local GPs is emphasized in the reports of both projects. The quality of the service that was delivered, however, seemed to win over public support in both cases.

Heaney and Paxton (1997) studied the Edinburgh unit over a 2-year period, during which time some 20 000 minor injuries patients were seen. Careful audit of notes showed that standards were met in 99 per cent of cases, and high levels of patient satisfaction were reported when two questionnaires were administered pre- and post-treatment. The only criticism from patients occurred when restrictive protocols meant that the nurse practitioners had to refer patients back to their GP or send them to an accident and emergency department elsewhere in the city. Patients found this difficult to understand, and the nurses found it very frustrating. The report makes no mention of the training the nurse practitioners had received, and once again it is clear that restrictive protocols are no substitute for proper educational preparation for the role.

The Horsham service was provided by nurse practitioners who had undergone a formal 3-month training programme (although no details are provided), supplemented by a further 12 weeks training in the accident and emergency department at Crawley. They had extensive protocols to guide their work, including drug protocols covering simple analgesia, antibiotics and tetanus toxoid injections.

The Mabrook and Dale (1998) report covers a full year, during which the emergency nurse practitioners saw 6944 new patients with minor injuries and reviewed 1611. They referred 234 patients to the main hospital accident and emergency department eight miles away due to the serious nature of their injuries. The largest group of referrals was to the physiotherapy service ($n = 352$), indicating the need to establish good links with the local physiotherapy department when setting up such a service. Audit of nurse practitioner radiographs revealed that out of 1945 requests, 760 (39 per cent) had fractures but 22 (2.9 per cent) of these fractures were missed and a further 57 false positives were recorded. No comment is made on the acceptability of this level of performance.

A patient satisfaction questionnaire was distributed to 313 patients and 269 returned. All but six patients stated that they were happy with the treatment and advice they had received, and with being treated by a nurse. The remaining six had no complaint about the nurse practitioners, but preferred to see a doctor. This study is, however, sparse on crucial details such as the nature of the nurse practitioner training and whether actual case notes were audited. It does give a detailed picture of the work undertaken, and concludes that with a good public education campaign and the provision of protocols that allow the nurse practitioner a large degree of autonomous practice, nurse practitioners can provide an effective minor injuries service. The alternative for the local population would be a substantial round trip of approximately 20 miles on congested roads to a major accident and emergency department.

If saving a round trip of 20 miles is worth while, then the study carried out by Chang *et al.* (1999) has even more significant mileage savings, as this study looked at the nurse practitioner role in a major rural emergency department in Australia. Once again, a picture of high levels of patient satisfaction is encountered. When treatment outcomes are compared with those achieved by medical staff, the nurse practitioners perform equally well.

The study looked at blunt trauma and wound management in a total of 232 patients allocated at random to either medical staff or nurse practitioners for their care. It probably included more severely injured patients than have been involved in some UK studies. The nurse practitioners enjoyed extensive autonomy in terms of radiography requests, prescribing and management of cases, and the study concluded that there was strong evidence and support for extending the nurse practitioner role into emergency departments in rural Australia.

Future developments

The innovative nature of the nurse practitioner role when applied in the unique situation of an accident and emergency department or emergency service opens up a range of exciting new possibilities. Radical approaches to service delivery are essential if we are to achieve the goal of renewing the NHS for a new century. Some of the following roles are being implemented, piloted or discussed at present; others are ideas to think about.

Adolescent drop-in health centre

There is increasing concern about teenage health in the UK, with issues such as the unacceptably high rate of pregnancies amongst teenage girls, drug use, eating disorders and young male suicides catching the headlines on a daily basis. Young people in the age range 12–18 years are often unwilling to attend health centres for a variety of reasons, such as the need to have a parent present, the fear of parents being informed even if they are not present, a feeling that doctors do not understand their problems, and the difficulty in gaining access at a time when the centre is open. The accident and emergency department is open 24 hours a day, and being seen by a neighbour or friend of a parent in accident and emergency is much easier to explain for the teenager, making a drop-in service more attractive. A nurse practitioner-led service catering specifically for the needs of teenagers could therefore be based in accident and emergency, and provide a new and valuable service that would reach a key group of people who are not currently accessing health care.

Nurse-led NHS walk-in centre

Work on establishing a network of walk-in centres began in 1999, and nurses are leading many of them. The model that seems to be emerging is one of heavy reliance upon software-driven protocols rather than allowing nurses more freedom to treat each patient on their merits. However, if the nursing staff employed do not possess the skills of a nurse practitioner and yet are expected to work in a 'first point of contact' role, this is hardly surprising, and we are encountering the same problem discussed already regarding minor injuries provision. As we write this book, there are no published evaluations of nurse-led walk-in centres. It is a reasonable hypothesis, however, that restrictive use of protocols will frustrate nurses and lead to a service that falls short of what was intended. An alternative hypothesis is that staffing walk-in centres with nurse practitioners who have the correct educational preparation, and who as a result have a greater degree of autonomy, will lead to a better service.

The emergency practitioner/paramedic

The growth in skills of ambulance personnel since the early 1980s has led to a major improvement in pre-hospital care and has undoubtedly contributed to the survival of many people who would otherwise have died. There is much debate at present within the ambulance service about the future of paramedic education and training. A strong argument exists for giving paramedics a deeper and wider theoretical base to underpin their existing clinical skills and also to facilitate significant expansion of their role in pre-hospital care. Many of the skills of the nurse practitioner are transferable to the paramedic, and a pilot scheme is under way at present in Cumbria involving a graduate nurse practitioner working as a paramedic, whilst discussions are taking place about recruiting paramedics to the undergraduate nurse practitioner degree course in that area. The emergency practitioner/paramedic could deliver more extensive emergency care in the pre-hospital situation than the current paramedic is allowed to. At the other end of the scale, it is possible that the emergency practitioner/paramedic could manage many 999 calls without taking the patient to accident and emergency. The use of nurse practitioner skills could lead to the patient being successfully managed at home or at the site of the incident and then taken home. Alternatively, referral for care to another health professional or social worker rather than a journey to accident and emergency would be more appropriate. In either situation the extra time spent with the patient could be offset by the benefits of a 'one-stop shop' approach to treatment, bypassing a lengthy wait in an accident and emergency department.

A nurse-led sexual assault service

A role that has developed recently in the USA is that of the sexual assault nurse examiner (SANE) based in the emergency department, who provides victims with comprehensive and holistic care from initial assessment and forensic examination, through treatment of acute injuries and on to long-term support and follow-up (Kagan-Krieger and Rehfeld, 2000). The physical and emotional needs of the victim are therefore paramount in this role, but evidence shows that it has also increased conviction rates. The nurse has to be able to carry out a full physical examination (including gathering forensic evidence), take a full medical history, diagnose and treat acute problems, and provide long-term emotional and psychological care – including referrals where needed for counselling. The role is very much that of a nurse practitioner providing holistic care to the victims of sexual crimes and in the process improving the chances of securing a conviction against the person responsible for the attack. The benefits are such that this is a role well worth investigation in the UK.

A nurse-led sports injury service

A high proportion of patients attending accident and emergency departments do so as a result of a sports injury. Sometimes their reception is affected by the view that it is a self-inflicted injury, which on a hectic Monday morning is not very welcome. Whether a knee injury results from falling awkwardly off a pavement, a road accident, stumbling on the bottom stair at home or from a tackle on the sports field, the treatment and advice given may be much the same. The differing forces at work in causing the injury and the different needs of the patient in terms of recovery may not be recognized. Consequently, serious sportsmen or women may feel that they do not receive an adequate service from the NHS. Playing sport undoubtedly has major health benefits as a result of enhanced levels of fitness, which justify treating sports injuries more seriously and appropriately. Some sports-oriented consultants do run specialist sports injury clinics, but many do not. Perhaps a nurse practitioner-led sports injury clinic, involving close liaison with the physiotherapy department, would provide the level of service that patients need. The benefits could include reduced workload on conventional accident and emergency services, better care for patients and a general enhancement of the fitness level of the population as a result of greater participation in sport.

A specialist nurse-led telephone advisory service

Marsden (1999) has described a nurse practitioner telephone triage service that operates in the ophthalmic accident and emergency department at Manchester Royal Eye Hospital. This should not be confused with NHS Direct. Apart from dealing with phone calls from the general public, the service offers advice to other health professionals such as practice nurses, occupational health nurses and nurses in other accident and emergency/minor injuries unit departments. The role described by Marsden (1999) illustrates that a nurse practitioner can work in a very specialist field, applying the general principles of nurse practitioner practice to the speciality in question. A nurse practitioner service such as this could become a regional or even a national resource, and need not be restricted to ophthalmology.

The examples cited above all depend upon the utilization of nurse practitioner skills, redrawing traditional role boundaries, and the unique interface with the community provided by the 24-hour accident and emergency service. The nurse practitioner role has tremendous potential in the provision of accident and emergency/minor injury services. However, the issue of correct educational preparation for the role is nowhere more important than in the front-line area of accident and emergency. In the author's own clinical experience, this is where a patient drives himself to hospital complaining of toothache, which turns out to be the referred pain of a myocardial infarction. Protocols and study days are no substitute for a well-educated graduate nurse practitioner who has a reasonable degree of autonomy in practice.

References

Allerton, J. and Justham, D. (2000a). Nurse practitioners and the Ottawa Ankle Rules: comparisons with medical staff in requesting X-rays for ankle injured patients. *A&E Nursing*, **8,** 110–15.

Allerton, J. and Justham, D. (2000b). A case-control study of the transit times through an accident and emergency department of ankle injured patients assessed using the Ottawa Ankle Rules. *A&E Nursing*, **8,** 148–54.

Barr, M., Johnston, D. and McConnell, D. (2000). Patient satisfaction with a new nurse practitioner service. *A&E Nursing*, **8,** 144–7.

Blunt, E. (1998). Role and productivity of the nurse practitioner in an urban emergency department. *J. Emergency Nursing*, **24(3),** 234–9.

Buchanan, L. and Powers, R. (1997). Establishing a nurse practitioner-staffed minor injuries area. *Nurse Practitioner*, **22,** 175–87.

Chang, E., Daly J., Hawkins, A. *et al.* (1999). An evaluation of the nurse practitioner role in a major rural emergency department. *J. Adv. Nursing*, **30(1),** 260–68.

Cole, F. (1998). Emergency nurse practitioner education: a United States perspective. *Emergency Nurse*, **6,** 12–14.

Dolan, B. (2000). *The Nurse Practitioner; Real World Research in Accident and Emergency*. Whurr.

Donnelly, L., Shifrin, T., Whitfield, L. and McIntosh, K. (2000). Make or break. *Health Services J.*, **3 Aug,** 12–17.

Heaney, D. and Paxton, F. (1997). Evaluation of a nurse-led minor injuries unit. *Nursing Standard*, **12(4),** 35–8.

Kagan-Krieger, S. and Rehfeld, G. (2000). The sexual assault nurse examiner. *Canadian Nurse*, **96(6),** 21–4.

Mabrook, A. and Dale, B. (1998). Can nurse practitioners offer a quality service? An evaluation of a year's work of a nurse-led minor injury unit. *J. A&E Med.*, **15,** 266–8.

Mann, C., Grant, J., Guly, H. and Hughes, P. (1998). Use of the Ottawa Ankle Rules by nurse practitioners. *J. A&E Med.*, **15(5),** 315–16.

Marsden, J. (1999). Expert decision-making: telephone triage in an ophthalmic accident and emergency department. *Nursing Times Res.*, **4(1),** 44–51.

Meek, S., Kendall. J., Porter, J. and Freij, R. (1998). Can accident and emergency nurse practitioners interpret radiographs? A multi-centre study. *J. A&E Med.*, **15(2),** 105–7.

Robinson, S. and Inyang, V. (1999). The nurse practitioner in emergency medicine – valuable but undefined. *Lancet*, **354,** 1319–26.

Sakr, M., Angus, J., Perrin, J. *et al.* (1999). Care of minor injuries by emergency nurse practitioners or junior doctors: a randomised controlled trial. *Lancet*, **354,** 1321–5.

Salt, P. and Clancy, M. (1997). Implementation of the Ottawa Ankle Rules by staff working in an accident and emergency department. *J. A&E Med.*, **14(6),** 363–5.

Tye, C., Ross, F. and Kerry, S. (1998). Emergency nurse practitioner services in major accident and emergency departments; a United Kingdom postal survey. *J. A&E Med.*, **15,** 31–4.

Walsh, M. (2000). The emerging role of the nurse practitioner in accident and emergency. *Emergency Nurse*, 7**(10),** 20–24.

Walsh, M., Crumbie, A. and Reveley, S. (1999). *Nurse Practitioners: Clinical Skills and Professional Issues*. Butterworth-Heinemann.

Yeats, W. B. (1910). The Coming of Wisdom with Time. In: *Selected Poetry* (N. Jeffares, ed.). Pan Books.

PART 3

Marketing, education and evaluation

9

EDUCATING THE NURSE PRACTITIONER

Alison Crumbie

Introduction

Nurse practitioners in hospital settings are relatively new to the UK. The role first emerged in accident and emergency settings and minor injuries units, but has now progressed to cover almost every speciality area in the hospital arena. The education of such a diverse group of higher level nurses who operate in both specialist and generalist areas poses quite a challenge for nurse educationalists. A further challenge is the absence of a clear definition of the role from the UKCC, resulting in local interpretation and a wide variety of approaches. Nurses who use the title 'nurse practitioner' have widely varying courses of preparation for their role, ranging from a few days of in-house training to a full Masters degree programme. This causes confusion for employers, colleagues, potential nurse practitioner students and, most importantly, patients. It is interesting to note that the Realising Specialist and Advanced Nursing Practice (RSANP) project was commissioned by the Department of Health in 1995, as at that time there was concern over a lack of shared understanding of the term 'nurse practitioner' and there was a wide variation in educational preparedness (Read and Roberts-Davis, 2000). Prior to this, Dowling *et al.* (1995) published an exploratory study into the boundaries between nurse practitioners and house officers. The authors concluded that there was a need for strategic issues to be considered, such as the development of appropriate education and the professional recognition of these developing roles. The issues raised by the Department of Health and Dowling *et al.* remain the same today. A lack of standardized educational preparation for nurse practitioners threatens patient safety and has the potential to halt the nurse practitioner movement in the UK. This chapter will explore the development of nurse practitioner education, and will consider the important elements that should be included in a curriculum for nurse practitioner students.

Development of nurse practitioner education

The educational preparation of nurse practitioners has its origins in the USA. In the 1960s, Henry Silver (a doctor) and Loretta Ford (a nurse) developed a programme of study for nurses who were working with children in the primary health care setting. Today in the USA there are a variety of nurse practitioner programmes across the country. It is possible to gain a nurse practitioner qualification through distance learning models, to study at Masters or post-Masters level, and to specialize in an area of practice such as adult, paediatric or elderly care. These courses are linked by standards that have been agreed by the National Task Force on Quality Nurse Practitioner Education facilitated by the National Organisation of Nurse Practitioner Faculties (NONPF).

The education and development of student nurse practitioners was first formalized in the United Kingdom by the Royal College of Nursing Institute of Advanced Nursing Education (RCNI). The course commenced at the RCNI in 1993. At this time the course was at diploma level and was firmly focused on primary care. In 1995 the course moved on to degree level. The RCNI went on to issue a statement that all nurse practitioners should be educated to at least first degree level (RCNI, 1997). During 1995 the RCNI course was franchised to other sites across the UK, and there was soon a network of educational providers for nurse practitioners. Simultaneously other courses were developing across the country, some using the title 'nurse practitioner' and others using a range of titles such as 'advanced clinical nurse'. These courses were offered at a variety of academic levels ranging from courses with no academic credit through to Masters level qualifications. Read and Roberts-Davis (2000) found that 29 higher education institutions across the UK responded to a postal survey on the educational provision of nurse practitioners during 1996. The courses that were available ranged from a fairly general approach through to very specific preparation for nurse practitioner or specialist practitioner practice. Some courses have been linked to the English National Board (ENB) Higher Award, and others have been linked to the ENB Developing Autonomous Practice Award (A33). In some areas the ENB A33 award is seen as sufficient for nurse practitioner preparation, and in other areas a culture has developed to lead nurses to believe that only a Masters degree is adequate. It can be seen that confusion and inconsistency still exists, and it is in this context that the report of the RSANP, *Preparing Nurse Practitioners for the 21st Century* (Read and Roberts-Davis, 2000), and the plan for accreditation of nurse practitioner courses by the RCNI (2000) is particularly welcome.

The RSANP report, *Preparing Nurse Practitioners for the 21st Century*, was based on a three-stage 'Delphi' research process. The aim was to reach a consensus amongst nurses in clinical practice, educators, purchasers, providers and representatives of statutory and professional bodies on the parameters and competencies for the nurse practitioner role. The results of the study identified agreed competencies that could be used as a measure of fitness for purpose for courses that aim to prepare nurse practitioners. The findings of the study enabled the development of suggested contents of the 'right' course for nurse practitioner education. In addition to the work of the RSANP project, a group of nurse practitioner education providers across the UK have been working on developing an accreditation system for nurse practitioner courses. The system includes 15 standards and a series of criteria that can be used to evaluate a programme of study for nurses to determine if it meets the agreed standard (Table 9.1). This chapter will examine both the proposed course content recommended by the RSANP project and the standards for nurse practitioner education provision proposed by the RCNI,

and will make suggestions as to how these frameworks can be integrated into a curriculum.

Educating the hospital nurse practitioner

In developing a curriculum for nurse practitioner students, it is important to remember that nurse practitioners are not defined by tasks or by technical competency. The first nurse practitioner graduates from the RCNI course in 1995 summed up the difference in their approach as, 'It's not what you do, it's the way that you do it'. The key to nurse practitioner practice is the highly developed skill of clinical decision making without reference to a doctor. It may be that some nurse practitioners will have to develop their technical skills in certain areas in order to function effectively in their particular area of practice; examples include the use of endoscopes in the colorectal clinic setting or the use of slit lamps in accident and emergency. However, the nurses are not defined by these tasks but by their ability to make autonomous decisions and to accept responsibility for those decisions. Underpinning this clinical decision-making skill is a broad base of knowledge focused on

Table 9.1 Standards and criteria for nurse practitioner courses

Joint working party between RCNI and NP education providers

The 15 standards with associated criteria are:
1. The higher education institution
2. Research and development
3. Meeting workforce requirements
4. Curriculum
5. Physical and learning resources
6. Recruitment and selection
7. Programme management
8. Leadership of the nurse practitioner programme
9. Staff resources
10. Staff development
11. Student support
12. Practice experience
13. Assessment
14. External examiners
15. Fitness for award

physiology, pathophysiology and pharmacology. There are also other highly developed clinical practice skills, including therapeutic communication, physical examination, consultation and history taking. Without this knowledge base the nurse is confined and restrained in practice, and the work in the clinical setting is more likely to be guided by strict protocols defined by medical colleagues and managers. A sound educational preparation for the nurse practitioner will unleash the nursing potential, allowing the practitioner to work effectively and efficiently in whatever setting is required.

There has been a tendency to define nurse practitioners as those nurses who accept patients with undifferentiated undiagnosed conditions; however, in the hospital setting nurse practitioners may work for the majority of the time with people who are presented to them with clearly defined conditions. There are nurse practitioners working in transplant services, fertility clinics and vascular surgery clinics, for example. In these situations the nurse practitioners are utilizing highly developed clinical decision-making skills to work with the patients presented to them, and they are able to go beyond the specialist area of practice to work with the patient in a holistic way. Take for example the nurse practitioner working in a rheumatology clinic, who will mostly be dealing with a very specific client group that presents with an already established clinical diagnosis. The highly developed skills of history taking and physical examination will allow the nurse practitioner to look beyond the musculoskeletal problem to notice other symptoms that the patient might have. If for example the client is also presenting with symptoms of depressed mood, the nurse practitioner would be able to go on to arrange for appropriate assessments and investigations to arrive at a diagnosis and then to arrange for appropriate treatment of the patient. Nurse practitioner skills allow the nurse to look beyond the immediately obvious, to scan the horizon for clues and to avoid missing important issues for the patient.

In addition to the clinical skills that are so much a part of the role, nurse practitioners are very involved in health promotion and patient education. Nurse practitioners in hospital settings have unique opportunities to work with patients on promoting their health and well-being. In accident and emergency units, for example, nurse practitioners interface with a greater number of young men than anywhere else in the health service. This is a perfect opportunity to offer health promotion messages, if appropriate and if the opportunity arises. Nurse practitioners working in a pre-operative assessment clinic may be the first health care professionals to pick up an opportunity to offer the patient some advice on smoking cessation. It is therefore important not to lose sight of this important component of the role when planning a curriculum.

Nurse practitioners have expanded the boundaries of their practice to include diagnostic reasoning, problem solving and consultation skills. The educational process for nurse practitioners therefore needs to address not only the practice elements of their clinical practice, but also higher level reasoning skills and the skills of reflection and analysis. Teaching and learning is a complex process which, combined with the clinical practice outcomes of nurse practitioner practice, takes on an additional dimension and depth (Chambers, 1999). The discussion above provides examples of the complexity of the role and the depth of analysis and clinical reasoning required in order to perform the role effectively. As well as developing the student's ability to think critically in the clinical situation, educational preparation for nurse practitioners should address the theory–practice gap and devise methods of ensuring that clinical skills such as physical examination are developed and utilized in the practice setting.

The RSANP executive summary provides a breadth of information on the role of the nurse practitioner. The RSANP team have identified the parameters of the nurse practitioner role, outlined the process involved in becoming a nurse practitioner, and identified core competencies for practice. Based on this they have made recommendations for the content of nurse practitioner courses. The recommendations are divided into four key areas: theoretical content; clinical practice skills content; teaching, learning and assessment strategies; and clinical practice management (Table 9.2).

The following discussion will consider these four key areas and link them to the accreditation system for nurse practitioner courses being piloted by the RCNI.

Table 9.2 RSANP four key areas for nurse practitioner courses

1. Theoretical content
2. Clinical practice skills content
3. Teaching, learning and assessment strategies and
4. Clinical practice management

Key elements of nurse practitioner courses

Theoretical content and clinical practice skills content

The RSANP group suggested that the theoretical content of a nurse practitioner course should include nursing, psychology/social psychology, ethics and law, research, biomedical sciences, clinical sciences and pharmacology. The clinical content should include history taking, physical examination, therapeutic communication, care planning and evaluation, and clinical decision making.

The recommendations related to the content of nurse practitioner courses identified by the RCN accreditation framework can be found in Table 9.3.

It is possible to see that the two recommendations are broadly the same. It is also possible to determine from these two lists that the educational preparation of nurse practitioners is complex and cannot be achieved with a few days of in-service training. The curriculum for

Table 9.3 The nurse practitioner programme

Content includes:
• Therapeutic nursing care:
 Comprehensive physical assessment of all body systems across the life span
 Health and disease, including physical, sociological, psychological and cultural aspects
• Epidemiology
• Pharmacology
• Research
 Organization and interpersonal skills, including group dynamics and counselling
 Legal and ethical issues
 Clinical decision making
 Professional role development
 Health promotion/disease prevention
• Communication in practice

nurse practitioner education should provide opportunities for the nurse to develop personally and professionally, to achieve higher level skills in clinical practice. The development of critical awareness and advanced problem-solving skills is essential. Without this breadth and depth of preparation we threaten the safety of our patients by placing in the clinical area nurses who are ill-prepared to deal with the demands of assessment, clinical decision making and diagnostic reasoning.

Development of clinical decision-making skills in the classroom poses an interesting challenge for the educator. Having utilized a thorough history-taking process, nurse practitioners should be able to consider multiple differential diagnoses for each patient presenting to them. They should be able to generate all of the potential differential diagnoses and then be able to engage in the process of clinical reasoning. The clinical reasoning process involves rejecting one hypothesis in favour of another, carrying out an appropriate physical examination and deciding upon the investigations necessary to confirm or disprove a diagnosis. Having developed a working diagnosis, the nurse practitioner should then be able to consider the treatment options available and be aware of the patient's values and beliefs in agreeing on a final decision for treatment, discharge or referral. It is clear that this complex activity relies upon a sound knowledge of a variety of subjects, including pathophysiology, pharmacology, communication skills, self-awareness and health promotion.

The skills required for engagement in this process include the ability to solve problems, take a thorough history and carry out a physical examination, and to be constantly open to alternative hypotheses as new information is revealed by the patient. A valuable tool for teaching this process includes the use of case studies in the classroom. The case study is offered to the students as 'the presenting patient', and they are supplied with the information available to them when a patient walks through the door or when they first meet. They are then asked to work through what history they might need to take and the physical examination they would perform, state which investigations they would like to arrange, and provide a rationale for each of these steps. Scenarios such as these can be worked through in the classroom in groups, with the decision-making process being discussed at each stage. If such discussions are linked to clinical decision-making models such as that of Barrows and Pickell (1991) or the stages models of problem solving (Hurst, 1993), this can be an example of truly linking theory to practice. The majority of students find these sessions to be extremely valuable. Texts that can help prepare students for such an approach include *Clinical Decision Making for Nurse Practitioners* (Robinson, 1998) and *The Symptom Sorter* (Hopcroft and Forte, 1999).

Teaching, learning and assessment strategies

In addition to a repertoire of physical, psychological and social skills, a nurse practitioner course should aim to help nurse practitioners to develop a sense of self-confidence, professional maturity and self-awareness throughout their course of study. Tutors and lecturers can work towards the latter factors through the appropriate use of teaching, learning and assessment strategies. The RSANP group suggested that teaching and learning strategies should include problem-based learning, reflection, critical incident journals and portfolios. Methods of assessment could include unseen and open-book examinations, multi-choice questionnaires and objective structured clinical examinations (OSCEs). The RCNI accreditation criteria state that:

… summative assessment schemes should include a rigorous, objective assessment of clinical competence using a variety of methods. The assessment should particularly address: history taking, physical examination, differential diagnosis, clinical decision making, and communication skills.

It is clear that both groups suggest that a variety of assessment strategies should be used in nurse practitioner programmes, and each institution should consider the options available to them in order to achieve the rigorous assessment of clinical competency.

The use of traditional methods of assessment is problematic when the complexity of the outcomes to be assessed on such a course is considered. Identification of the appropriate method of assessment for nurse practitioner students is essential, as the assessment process has a great impact upon the learning experience of the students. Nicklin and Lankshear (1995) suggest that it is important to consider the purpose of the assessment process. The assessment of nurse practitioners should aim to protect the public, judge the level of student achievement, monitor student progress, predict the future behaviour of the nurse and motivate the students, and can also be used to measure the effectiveness of the teaching. Nurse practitioners do not engage in a task-oriented approach to patient care; instead they approach the patient holistically. The assessment of nursing practice should therefore mirror this emphasis by moving away from teacher domination to student participation. Knowles (1990) would agree with this statement, as he commented that the education of adults is a process of active inquiry rather than a passive receipt of transmitted content. The nurse practitioner educator must then consider methods of enhancing the active involvement of the students in the learning process, and one such method might be the development of a portfolio.

The portfolio of learning

The andragogical approach to teaching and learning would suggest that adult learners resent and resist situations in which they feel that others are imposing their will on them (Knowles, 1990). A portfolio can provide the flexibility of structure for students to develop a personal approach to the assessment process. The teacher in this case then merely facilitates that process, guided by the learning outcomes of the course, the competencies of a nurse practitioner and individual students' identified learning needs. The portfolio can be used to hand the control back to student nurse practitioners by allowing them to choose how they are going to approach the narratives and what evidence they are going to provide to prove that they meet the learning outcomes. One method of formalizing this approach is to request that portfolio development be guided by learning contracts. Learning contracts enable students to take control of their own learning, and they can therefore make their own assessment of whether their aims have been achieved (Alavi and Cooke, 1995) (Table 9.4).

The foundation of the portfolio should be reflective practice, so that individual students

Table 9.4 Guidelines for developing a learning contract

---

1. Assessment:
   - What skills need to be developed?
   - What aspects of the role need developing?
2. Planning:
   - What are the intended learning outcomes?
   - What strategies and resources can you use to achieve these outcomes?
   - Who will evaluate performance, and what criteria will be used?
3. Negotiation:
   - Discuss and negotiate the learning contract with facilitator and course tutor
4. Implementation:
   - Identification of actual learning outcomes achieved
   - Refer to intended learning outcomes
   - Action plan for future

---

are constantly incorporating new knowledge with experiences from clinical practice. This can be quite challenging for students, as not only are they required to produce a highly complex piece of written work demonstrating their ability to analyse critically and to link theory to practice, but also to use the skill of reflective practice to incorporate their experiences from practice within their written work. An evaluation of the nurse practitioner students' experience of portfolio development was carried out at St Martin's College in 1999 (Crumbie, 1999). The students were asked what was the best part of the experience of writing a portfolio for the nurse practitioner degree course, and what was the worst part of the experience. Most of the students stated that the worst part was starting it, and the best part was handing it in! However, there were several other comments that we found illuminating and have helped to inform the way the portfolio is used with subsequent groups of students. One student stated that the best part of the experience was 'feeling enthusiastic about the nurse practitioner role', and another student stated the best part was 'ending and realizing what I had achieved ... unaware of what one does until asked to sit and write about it'. The worst part of the experience for one student was 'cross-referencing the information as it applied to various sections', and another was 'focusing on what was required

and not what I wanted to say'. These comments reflect the problem of the complexity of the portfolio and also the tendency of students to feel that they have to fit the 'ideal portfolio'. In fact the guidelines on portfolio development given to the students are very flexible, and the students are encouraged to negotiate with the tutors to develop their individual style and reflect their unique working situations. It is possible that some students may not believe that this is the case, and they still search for the 'formula' or 'recipe' for production of assessed work.

Students may find an exam or a 3000-word assignment easier than a portfolio as they are provided with a template for their work which, if followed, can guarantee their success. This 'canned' approach to assignment writing discourages critical thinking (Sorrell *et al.*, 1997). A portfolio, however, challenges students to think creatively, to solve problems, and to develop their own approach to the challenge of presenting such a personal piece of work. Many assignments designed to examine student achievement are not specifically designed to foster particular skills of thinking. The portfolio does, however, require the student to engage in problem solving in order to compile the piece of work. In many ways this mirrors clinical practice more effectively than other forms of written assessment.

One potential problem with the portfolio is the need to gain experience in the clinical setting to support the reflections and evidence in the work. Cayne (1995) commented that those students who find themselves in clinical areas that are not conducive to innovative practice have difficulty in collecting evidence for their portfolios. It is not uncommon for student nurse practitioners to be restricted in their practice until they have completed the course, particularly in areas where there is a lack of familiarity with the role. This restriction makes it extremely difficult for students to practise their developing skills, and therefore they may experience great difficulty in generating the evidence for their work. This particular problem provides evidence of the need to have a supportive network in the student nurse practitioner's place of practice; without the support and encouragement of colleagues and employers the role will not flourish and the student will experience difficulty in progressing on the course.

Reflective practice

Knowles (1990) suggests that adult learners come into education with a whole history of prior experience, which can be problematic as they may have biases and habits, or it can be enriching and relevant to the current educational experience. It is important therefore to develop the skill of reflective practice, and this in turn can enhance self-awareness and provide an opportunity to develop new perspectives on old ways of knowing. Reflective practice and critical incidents can be used in a variety of forms throughout the programme. The students may be asked to reflect on their first ever physical examination, and to compare this with an examination carried out one year later. Critical incidents can be used to allow the student to examine key elements of their role in some depth, and they can be used as narratives in their portfolios.

Atkins and Murphy (1993) state that reflection as a learning tool is a necessary process in professional education. These authors point out that practice is central to nursing, and if learning is to occur from practice, reflection is vital. Mackintosh (1998) points out, however, that reflection is a term that is confused and ill-defined. Some authors have attempted to define reflection. Atkins and Murphy (1993) state that there is a lack of definition and clarity relating to the concept of reflective practice. Boyd and Fales (1983) suggest that:

… reflective learning is the process of internally examining and exploring an issue of concern, triggered by experience which creates and clarifies meaning in terms of self and which results in a changed conceptual perspective.

Boud *et al.* (1985) state that:

… reflection in the context of learning is a generic term for those intellectual and affective activities in which individuals engage to explore their experiences in order to lead to new understandings and appreciations.

The two definitions identify a process of personal exploration followed by a changed perspective.

Based on a review of the literature and the two definitions outlined above, Atkins and Murphy (1993) state that there are three stages to the reflective process, which begins with an awareness of uncomfortable feelings and thoughts, leads on to a critical analysis of feelings and knowledge, and finally results in a new perspective. This is not simply a linear model, as the three stages are integrated; however, it does provide a useful tool for analysis of reflection. Reflection requires the practitioner to think about the experience and to analyse events critically, leading to changed perspectives; thus each situation is regarded as a unique event, and the care delivered is less likely to become routine.

Nurse practitioners deal with patients and their families in complex clinical situations. Clinical problems are indeterminate, and often have elements of uncertainty and conflict. Donald Schön (1987) pointed out that the scientific approach to problem solving known as 'technical rationality' did not necessarily address the complexity of clinical problem solving. Technical rationality is based on the assumption that a problem can be identified or that the ends of the problem are fixed. It represents a pure 'applied science' view of professional practice with a focus on the acquisition of generic competencies of systematic problem solving (Greenwood, 1993). Schön (1987) suggested that technical problem solving needed to be placed within the broader context of reflective enquiry or reflective practice in order to right the wrongs of technical rationality.

Learning to become an effective practitioner is not simply a process of acquiring skills, it requires personal deconstruction and reconstruction involving a process of empowerment, enlightenment and emancipation (Johns, 1995). This process involves the practitioner having the courage to develop self-awareness, to take action to change the self and develop a vision of who he or she needs to be to achieve effective and desirable practice. Clearly the aim of reflective practice is to provide a broad context for clinical problem solving and therefore to enhance the practitioner's clinical practice.

Lyons (1999) describes methods of engaging students in exercises to develop their descriptive writing skills and therefore enhance their ability to reflect. Mackintosh (1998) states that journals, reflective diaries, reflective workshops and critical incident analysis are all techniques that have been used to engage the student in reflection. Heath (1998) points out that it is a mistake to equate the skills of reflection only with academic skills. She suggests that clinical ability is also a necessary skill, as the novice may have difficulty in seeing beyond the tasks and therefore will have difficulty in engaging in the reflective process. It is particularly valuable to explore the skills required to engage in reflective practice, as the students clearly need to develop these skills before the full benefit of reflection as a learning tool can be realized.

Reflective practice is used widely in nursing education, and in many curricula it forms the basis of assessment. Mackintosh (1998) points out that the concept remains poorly defined and, if reflection is to be used to assess students, a uniform method of instrumentation should be used. There is no clear guidance relating to the assessment of the content of the reflection or the process of reflective practice (Andrews *et al.*, 1998). This is particularly important in a course that is focused on clinical ability, as the students need to display clinical competency in assessed work. If one of the aims of reflective practice is that students should learn from examples of poor practice, then the content of the reflection needs to be assessed with caution. Newell (1992) criticizes reflection for its reliance on one person's ability to recall events. Johns (1998), however, defends this, as he states that it is not the accuracy of the reflection that is important, rather it is the meaning that the practitioner gives to the situation. If the practitioner has distorted the facts for some reason, this is a factor which in itself it is important to understand.

Several authors (Andrews *et al.*, 1998; Mackintosh, 1998) state that there is a lack of empirical evidence to indicate that engaging in reflection changes practice or improves patient outcomes. Benefits to individuals engaging in clinical practice have been demonstrated (Butterworth *et al.*, 1997), and this links with Johns (1995), as he states that the purpose of reflective practice is to enable the practitioner to access, understand and learn through lived experiences, and therefore to take congruent action towards developing effectiveness within the context of what is understood as desirable clinical practice. Models of reflection such as the Gibbs cycle (Gibbs, 1988) based on Kolb's (1984) experiential learning cycle and Johns (1995) model of structured reflection can be used in clinical teaching and the assessment of practice, but should be used with caution and an awareness of the limitation of the use of reflective practice in the classroom.

The objective structured clinical examination

One method of making a direct link between examinations and clinical practice is the use of objective structured clinical examinations (OSCE). Selby *et al.* (1995) describe an OSCE as 'a circuit of assessment stations, where a range of practical clinical skills are assessed by an examiner using a previously determined, objective marking scheme'. The OSCE involves a series of 'stations' where a student consults with a patient whilst being assessed by an examiner. The stations can be focused on history taking, physical examination skills, communication skills or management of emergency situations. As the stations are piloted and evaluated for their validity and reliability, it is important to remember that there are three other potential variables in an OSCE station – the patient, the examiner and the student. When setting up an OSCE examination, the assessment team must ensure that the examiners are well trained in their role and that the patients are consistent in their stories.

At St Martin's College we have found that the OSCE has an enormous impact on the students' experience of the whole course. We frequently use OSCE scenarios in the classroom to help the students to engage in problem-based learning. We have also discovered that students find the OSCE stations a useful means to focus their energies in learning sets, and this enables them to provide feedback to one another. This seems to foster mutual support and encouragement. We examine the students with a short OSCE in their first year of study on the nurse practitioner course. The mini OSCE involves two stations: one physical examination and one history-taking station. This ensures that there is a focus on the all-important nurse practitioner skills at the start of the course. We have evaluated the mini OSCE, and found that the majority of students appreciate this kind of assessment at an early stage in their course. Most of the students report that going through the OSCE increases their confidence and it helps them to be sure that they are carrying out their examinations appropriately. There is no doubt, however, that going through an OSCE is an extremely stressful experience, and in their final year the students on the St Martin's course have to complete an OSCE of 10 stations.

The final OSCE examines a greater breadth and depth of knowledge than the examination in the first year. At this stage the students are expected to interpret their findings and make decisions about the plan of care for the patient. The structure of the St Martin's OSCE is three physical examination stations, three history-taking stations, three communication stations and one written station. The written station allows us to examine areas of clinical practice that would otherwise be difficult to replicate with a patient in the false situation of the examination. Examples of this might be a patient suffering a hypoglycaemic attack or an epileptic fit, examples of dermatological lesions, or assessment of a patient with a head injury. An example of a full OSCE for hospital nurse practitioners is given in Table 9.5.

There are other methods of rigorously assessing clinical competency, including visits to the student's place of practice by outside assessors, conducting a full head-to-toe physical examination, and the use of videos. There have also been other approaches to the OSCE process that include the use of integrated stations which involve taking a history, carrying out a physical examination and offering the patient advice based on the findings. Whichever approach is used, it is important that the tool is valid and reliable and that the method of assessment accurately

reflects the student's competency. There is no room for error in the assessment of clinical competency. It would be a grave mistake to fail a student who was actually competent, and, even more importantly, it would be negligent to allow an incompetent student to pass the OSCE. It is therefore of paramount importance that whichever tool is used to assess the student, it has been piloted, tested, and deemed to be valid and reliable. The focus on assessment of clinical practice links to clinical practice management, the fourth key area in nurse practitioner courses identified by the RSANP group.

Other forms of assessment

The RCNI standards suggest that a variety of approaches to assessment should be used in nurse practitioner courses. There are many methods of assessing students, including the use of audio and video-tapes in practice, the presentation of seminars and case studies in the classroom, written assignments and reports, and formal examinations. Formal examinations can be useful in assessing the student's understanding of pathophysiology and pharmacology. Nurse practitioners in practice have ready access to copies of the *British National Formulary* (2000), and it therefore seems reasonable that they should be allowed to have a copy of it with them during a pharmacology examination. Multi-choice examination questions can be used to examine

Table 9.5 Example of an objective structured clinical examination

Scenario	Skill being tested
Patient with a history of a cough	History-taking
Examination of respiratory system	Physical examination
Patient has fallen and hit her head	Communication and giving advice
Patient complains of being tired all the time	History taking
Photograph of a patient with eczema	Knowledge of eczema and ability to describe the lesions using appropriate terminology
Patient presents with ankle pain	History taking, communication and advice
Examination of the back	Physical examination
Patient being examined in clinic and found to smoke 20 cigarettes each day	Communication and giving advice in relation to smoking cessation
Examination of abdomen	Physical examination
Patient is experiencing anxiety with panic attacks	Communication skills in relation to patients with mental health problems

some of the hard facts in physiology and pathophysiology; however this would need to be combined with an assignment that allows the student the opportunity to link the pathophysiology to a patient in the clinical setting. Nurse practitioners work in clinical practice, and therefore all of their assessments should make sense to them in the clinical setting.

Clinical practice management

Clinical practice is the cornerstone of nurse practitioner role development. NONPF recommend that students achieve a minimum of 500 hours in clinical practice during the course of their study to become nurse practitioners. This recommendation may vary between courses; however, it seems reasonable to suggest that students should be able to practise nurse practitioner skills on at least half a day of each week during the course of study. In reality, if the students are on a part-time course they will gradually incorporate the nurse practitioner skills into their current role as the course progresses, and will far exceed half a day a week of practice. For students who are on a full-time nurse practitioner course, exposure to the clinical setting must be an integral component of the programme. The RCNI standards include a criterion stating that 'nurse practitioner students have access to patient populations specific to their area of practice, sufficient in number and variability to ensure that the programme learning outcomes are met'. This raises the questions of how the clinical practice will be supervised, and how the safety of patients will be ensured during the period of training and education.

One method of supervising the work of nurse practitioner students has been to enlist the assistance of medical practitioners in the student's area of clinical practice; this person will then become the student's facilitator. The facilitator has the responsibility of ensuring that the student develops physical examination skills in practice and gains a breadth of clinical experience during the time spent on the course. The facilitator's role is not to be confused with being responsible for assessment of the student; rather, the aim of the facilitator is to work with the student to ensure that they cover the clinical competencies listed in the nurse practitioner competency file. Summative assessment of the students rests with the nurse practitioner course team, and this reduces some of the tension that might exist between the facilitator and the student.

It may be possible to enlist the assistance of an experienced nurse practitioner in facilitating the student's experience in clinical practice. In many programmes in the USA, a nurse practitioner faculty exists that can help the students gain the necessary clinical experience during the course. In the UK, however, there are very few appropriately qualified and experienced hospital nurse practitioners to help guide the development of students. In many ways there is a great advantage in working with both medical practitioners and nurse mentors. As we enter the twenty-first century the role of the hospital nurse practitioner is moving into uncharted territory. The more members of the health care team we can engage in the process the more successful these pioneering nurses are likely to be.

Whoever is involved in the facilitation of clinical experience, it can be helpful to guide and focus the direction of the experience gained during the nurse practitioner course. The RSANP team stated that clinical practice should be integral to the programme, should form a substantial component of it, and should be planned with clear objectives. Nurse practitioners work in a breadth of specialities in hospital settings, and all of the students will enter the course with varied experience and a wealth of past experience in clinical practice. It is clear then that no two students are likely to require the exact same clinical experience during the nurse practitioner course. A dermatological nurse practitioner might feel that his or her assessment of skin lesions is well developed, but may lack experience of gynaecological assessment. However, a gynaecological nurse practitioner might feel that his or her knowledge of the assessment of skin lesions is poorly developed, and whilst capable of adequate gynaecological examinations may want to develop them even further. In such situations the use of learning contracts can help students to identify to their knowledge gaps and plan, with their facilitator, approaches to their learning to help address these gaps. This exemplifies the andragogical approach to teaching and learning, and acknowledges the unique experience and learning needs of each student on the nurse practitioner programme.

Conclusion

Earlier in this book (see Chapter 4) we noted that student hospital nurse practitioners identified that in-house training did not adequately prepare them for their role in clinical practice. The students identified the need for a formal approach to education to provide a breadth and depth to their study that could not be provided in their place of clinical practice. We also noted that the students identified the need to explore new ways of problem solving in clinical practice. In Chapter 4 we noted that knowledge is a resource to nurse practitioners, and in Chapter 2 we identified the need to integrate medical skills into a nursing model to underpin nurse practitioner practice. It is clear from these comments and from the discussion outlined in this chapter that nurse practitioners require formal education to provide the foundation for their clinical practice. The formal education should at least meet the standards outlined by the RCNI accreditation unit and address the four key areas identified by the RSANP group. Anything less than this is a disservice to our patients and will diminish the standard and quality that should be associated with the title 'nurse practitioner'.

References

Alavi, C. and Cooke, M. (1995). Assessing problem-based learning. In: *Problem-based Learning in a Health Sciences Curriculum* (C. Alavi, ed.), pp. 126–40. Routledge.

Andrews, M., Gidman, J. and Humphreys, A. (1998). Reflection: does it enhance professional nursing practice? *Br. J. Nursing*, **7(7)**, 413–17.

Atkins, S. and Murphy, K. (1993). Reflection: a review of the literature. *J. Adv. Nursing*, **18**, 1188–92.

Barrows, H. S. and Pickell, G. C. (1991). *Developing Clinical Problem-Solving Skills: A Guide to More Effective Diagnosis and Treatment*. Norton Medical Books.

Boud, D., Keogh, R. and Walker, D. (1985). *Reflection: Turning Experience into Learning*. Kegan Page.

Boyd, E. M. and Fales, A. W. (1983). Reflective learning: key to learning from experience. *J. Humanistic Psychol.*, **23(2)**, 99–117.

Butterworth, C. A., Carson, J., White, E. *et al.* (1997). *It's Good to Talk. An Evaluation Study in England and Scotland*. University of Manchester.

Cayne, J. V. (1995). Portfolios: a developmental influence? *J. Adv. Nursing*, **21**, 395–405.

Chambers, N. (1999). Close encounters: the use of critical reflective analysis as an evaluation tool in teaching and learning. *J. Adv. Nursing*, **29(4)**, 950–57.

Crumbie, A. (1999). The portfolio as a form of assessment for nurse practitioners. Sixth International Nurse Practitioner Conference Presentation, August 1999.

Dowling, S., Barrett, S. and West, R. (1995). With nurse practitioners, who needs house officers? *Br. Med. J.*, **311**, 309–13.

Gibbs, G. (1988). *Learning by Doing: A Guide to Teaching and Learning Methods*. Further Education Unit.

Greenwood, J. (1993). Reflective practice: a critique of the work of Argyris and Schön. *J. Adv. Nursing*, **18**, 1183–7.

Heath, H. (1998). Reflection and patterns of knowing in nursing. *J. Adv. Nursing*, **27**, 1054–9.

Hopcroft, K. and Forte, V. (1999). *The Symptom Sorter*. Radcliffe Medical Press.

Hurst, K. (1993). *Problem Solving in Nursing Practice*. Scutari Press.

Johns, C. (1995). Framing learning through reflection within Carper's fundamental ways of knowing in nursing. *J. Adv. Nursing*, **22**, 226–34.

Johns, C. (1998). Opening the doors of perception. In: *Transforming Nursing Through Reflective Practice* (C. Johns and D. Freshwater, eds), pp. 1–20. Blackwell Science.

Knowles, M. (1990). *The Adult Learner: A Neglected Species*, 4th edn. Gulf Publishing.

Kolb, D. (1984). *Experiential Learning: Experience as a Source of Learning and Development*. Prentice-Hall.

Lyons, J. (1999). Reflective education for professional practice: discovering knowledge from experience. *Nurse Ed. Today*. **19**, 29–34.

Mackintosh, C. (1998). Reflection: a flawed strategy for the nursing profession. *Nurse Ed. Today*, **18**, 553–7.

Newell, R. (1992). Anxiety, accuracy and reflection: the limits of professional development. *J. Adv. Nursing*, **17**, 1326–33.

Nicklin, P. and Lankshear, A. (1995). The principles of assessment. In: *Teaching and Assessing in Nursing Practice: An Experiential Approach*, 2nd edn (P. Nicklin and N. Kenworthy, eds), pp. 68–80. Scutari Press.

Read, S. and Roberts-Davis, M. (2000). *Preparing Nurse Practitioners for the 21st Century*. Executive Summary from the Report of the Project 'Realising Specialist and Advanced Nursing Practice: Establishing the Parameters of and Identifying the Competencies for "Nurse Practitioner" Roles and Evaluating Programmes of Preparation (RSANP)'. Sheffield University.

Robinson, D. (1998). *Clinical Decision Making for Nurse Practitioners*. Lippincott.

Royal College of Nursing Institute (2000). *Standards and Criteria for RCN Accreditation of Nurse Practitioner (NP) Programmes Offered in Collaborating Higher Education Institutions (HEIs): A Discussion Document*. RCN.

Schön, D. (1987). *Educating the Reflective Practitioner*. Basic Books.

Selby, C., Osman, L., Davis, M. and Lee, M. (1995). How to do it: set up and run an objective structured clinical exam. *Br. Med. J.*, **310**, 1187–90.

Sorrell, J. M., Brown, H. N., Cipriano Silva, M. and Kohlenberg, E. M. (1997). Use of portfolios for interdisciplinary assessment of critical thinking outcomes of nursing students. *Nursing Forum*, **32(4)**, 12–23.

10

MARKETING THE ROLE OF THE NURSE PRACTITIONER

Chris Batten and Alison Crumbie

I keep six honest serving-men
(They taught me all I knew);
Their names are What and Why and When
And How and Where and Who.
          The Elephant's Child, by Rudyard Kipling

Introduction

Now isn't marketing all about advertising, promotion and selling? Well yes ... but that's not all. We will be inviting you to think about marketing on a number of levels – first, as a framework for evaluating the services you offer and asking yourself if they best meet the needs of your clients; secondly, at a more strategic level, where marketing frameworks will allow you to plan how to position yourself within the health care setting; and thirdly, as a way of thinking, to help you deal more effectively with the ever-increasing changes and pressures on the nurse practitioner role.

The aim of this chapter is to enable you to consider everything from the macro-environment in which you practise, right down to daily interactions with patients. We hope that by considering your practice with a marketing orientation you will be better equipped to enhance the services offered. As the Kipling quote suggests, if you're not asking the questions, you're unlikely to find the answers.

Definitions of marketing

The Chartered Institute of Marketing in the UK states that 'marketing is the management process responsible for identifying, anticipating and satisfying customer requirements profitably' (Chartered Institute of Marketing, 2000). Young (1995) provides a simpler overview of marketing within the context of nursing as 'solving customers' problems', whilst McDermott (1996) embellishes the Chartered

Institute of Marketing definition further to say that 'it is concerned with managing the exchange that takes place between those that provide the service and those that receive it'. We are not convinced that any of these are adequate; Young is placing an emphasis on satisfying patient needs, whilst McDermott is talking about the broader health care setting in which you operate. In the end a marketing strategy will need to incorporate both of these elements. A marketing approach that incorporates this broader perspective is known as 'relationship marketing'.

Relationship marketing

Nurse practitioners are not alone in struggling to make the connection from selling washing powder on the television to satisfying the needs of their patients. Marketing as an academic discipline began with fast-moving consumer goods in the USA in the 1950s, and hence has long been associated with supermarket goods. Indeed, it is only in the last 15 years that a growing body of literature has begun to interpret this traditional marketing theory and relate it to the provision of professional services such as those offered by nurse practitioners. A key aspect of the bridge between the two is the concept of relationship marketing, and it is this that will inform the basis of our approach in this chapter. Relationship marketing focuses on creating and maintaining long-term relationships with clients and all other relevant stakeholders in health care provision. For a nurse practitioner, for example, this might include not only individual patients and their families, but also the hospital management, consultants, other health care staff, community staff, equipment suppliers, drug companies and the government.

Relationship marketing suggests that nurse practitioners need to develop and enhance relationships with each of these groups in order to maximize the effectiveness of their role. However, arriving at the stunning conclusion that 'it's all about relationships' is probably not going to amaze nursing professionals around the country. It is, however, the umbrella concept that covers and permeates all of the detail that follows – a point that is well worth remembering as we delve into the detail of the following analysis, planning and implementation tools.

Marketing models

Our first forays into marketing revealed a bewildering array of acronyms. Consider the glossary in Table 10.1, which is indicative of

Table 10.1 A Services Marketing glossary

Term	Meaning
The four Marketing Ps – also known as the Marketing Mix	Used to structure the planning and implementation of marketing activities under the headings of: Product (the total service package provided to patients) Price (obviously what it costs, but this can also be seen as value) Place (how and where you make your services available to the public) Promotion (how you communicate with existing/potential patients) Other Ps that are often considered in Services Marketing include: People (the knowledge, skills and abilities of you/your colleagues) Processes (the interactions critical to the effective delivery of services) Physical environment (the feel and appearance of your clinic, etc.)
SWOT analysis	A structure to distil data from a strategic audit of your practice/organization that is divided into Strengths and Weaknesses (internal) and Opportunities and Threats (external)
PLC	Describes the Product Life Cycle (or Service offering in our context) from inception to completion, involving the four distinct stages of: Introduction >> Growth >> Maturity >> Decline
STEP analysis	Four areas of macro-environmental analysis (refer to Table 10.2, page 121) grouped as: Sociological/Technological/Economic/Political
Market	All existing and potential users of your service(s) – e.g. all patient groups
Industry	All providers of services similar to your own – e.g. the health care industry
Sector	Specific groups of services – e.g. primary care groups
Segmentation	Identifying a group of users with common needs or characteristics – e.g. people suffering from asthma in a rural area
Targeting	Focusing your marketing mix to address a specific market segment – e.g. encouraging men over 50 to have their cholesterol and blood pressure checked
Positioning	Your place in the industry relative to other providers according to various criteria (such as friendliness, professionalism, efficiency, cost, access, hygiene, etc.) as perceived by the patient
CRM	Client Relationship Marketing/Management
Services Marketing	As distinct from marketing goods or products primarily because services rely on people to deliver them
Ansoff's product-market growth matrix	A 2 × 2 matrix that describes four distinct marketing strategies, with Existing–New Markets along one axis and Existing–New Products along the other axis
Branding	How people recognize and feel about your services and/or organization

marketers' predilection for analytical models with confounding names. Our view is that they all have a part to play in understanding your practice from a marketing perspective, so the real challenge is knowing the order in which to use them and how they fit into the bigger marketing picture.

To help with this, we have created the model shown in Figure 10.1 as a marketing flowchart, and we will go on to explore each box in turn. In order to understand the reason why we have ordered Figure 10.1 – and therefore this chapter – in the way we have, consider the following links:

- The *why* – i.e. using the findings from the internal and external audits to inform your strategic planning decisions
- The *where* – i.e. the picture of the future embodied in the vision and mission

- The *what* – i.e. the most important goals that describe what you are trying to change and achieve
- The *how* – i.e. a detailed plan of how you and your colleagues are going to meet those important goals
- The *when* – i.e. the measurable actions associated with implementing your plan.

And, just to keep Kipling happy, the *who* is you.

Marketing analysis, planning, implementation and review

Starting the process of writing a strategy for your practice or organization without gathering relevant information first is a little like

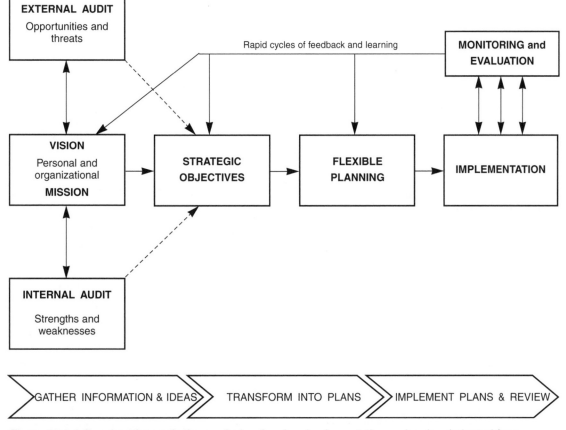

Figure 10.1 A flowchart for marketing analysis, planning, implementation and review (adapted from Watts, 1996).

diagnosing patients' conditions without knowing anything about them. You need the data in order to make considered decisions based on sound evidence. For that reason we recommend that your marketing plan should begin with gathering insight and perspectives both within and outside your health care setting.

The acronym SWOT (Strengths, Weaknesses, Opportunities and Threats) is often used as shorthand for the type of analysis you need to undertake at this stage. SWOT describes both the internal audit (the strengths and weaknesses of your organization) and the external audit (the opportunities and threats within the broader macro-environment in which you operate) referred to in Figure 10.1. We will consider each in turn.

The external audit

If ever you need a reason to investigate the macro-environment in which you operate, then just consider the impact that successive governments had on the organization and delivery of health care in the UK during the 1990s. Also referred to as environmental scanning (Brownlie, 1988), the question we are trying to address is, *what external factors will impact significantly on your practice in the future?* A number of frameworks have been put forward to help in answering this question, including the early work of Kast and Rosenwieg (1974; cited in Brownlie, 1988), in which they identified nine areas for study and analysis (the so-called STEP analysis is a simplified version of this; see Table 10.1). The key to using these frameworks is to gather all the information you can in order to identify trends that could impact upon you and your patients. Table 10.2 provides an example of the types of questions you should be asking in each of these nine areas.

In addition to drawing on your own experience, there are a number of useful sources from which you can glean this type of information in relation to the health care market. They include:

- The National Health Service (www.nhs. org.uk)
- The National Institute of Clinical Excellence (www.nice.org.uk)
- Medical and nursing media (e.g. *Nursing Standard*, www.nursing-standard.co.uk; *British Medical Journal*, www.bmj.com etc)
- The National Institute for Clinical Excellence (www.nice.org.uk)
- The Department of Health (www.doh. gov.uk.org)
- The Royal College of Nursing (www.rcn. org.uk)
- Community Health Councils (www.achcew. org.uk)
- Colleagues, patients and allied health practitioners
- Local health authorities
- Local colleges and universities
- Public libraries
- Voluntary agencies, not-for-profit organizations and charities.

Having begun to compile a list of factors that will impact upon your practice, you should then begin the process of prioritizing them in order of importance as well as considering whether they comprise an opportunity or a threat. The main difficulty in identifying these trends is in thinking forward, based on current information. Those who predicted the demise of the cinema when video became popular were as wrong as those who were investing in typewriters at the beginning of the personal computer evolution.

Within our industry, examples of how to think through future developments based on current information include the following aspects:

- *Legal*: a new court ruling on the role of the nurse practitioner could have an impact upon the way in which we are able to develop advanced nursing roles in the future. For example, what if a nurse had been involved in a legal case where the diagnosis and treatment carried out in the minor injuries unit by that nurse was questioned in court? Let's say the court then ruled that it was acceptable for nurses to carry out such activities so long as they were appropriately qualified and educated. This ruling would have an impact upon the activity of nurse practitioners thereafter. At the governmental level, the degree to which a nurse practitioner can prescribe certain medications is dependent upon the Medicines Act (HMSO, 1968). Recent consultation documents (DoH, 2000a) have suggested that nurse prescribing may be rolled out to include

Table 10.2 Analysis of external factors

Cultural	What are the changing cultural norms of your region and how will they impact on your service to patients? One example would be the implications of a patient's religion and how you can best treat them
Technological	How might technological advances impact upon your organization? Will technology provide you with new knowledge or changed ways of operating in your environment? What technological capability do you have now, and how does this compare with what is possible?
Educational	What is the current norm for training and education in your profession, and what is the trend for training professionals in your industry in the future? Do you have access to a large pool of fully qualified nurse practitioners and a plentiful supply of doctors and consultants? If the population continues to become more health literate, how will nursing professionals continue to add value?
Political	What is the political climate at the local, regional and national level? What impact is the current government having upon the health services you provide? What impact will a change of government have on your practice?
Legal	Are there any legal restraints on developing practice in your organization? Does legislation support your practice, or do you have to practise defensively as the law does not enable you to realize the full potential of the workforce in your organization? Do you have access to a legal team to advise on developments in practice? Does the United Kingdom Central Council (UKCC) recognize and protect the titles used by nurses in your organization?
Environmental	The depleted ozone layer over Australia led to a dramatic rise in the diagnosis and treatment of skin cancer, which initially caught many health professionals by surprise. What are the ecological trends that will impact on your patient population over the coming years? Will access to road transport limit your ability to deliver an outreach service? Will government guidelines on the ecological efficiency of your hospital affect your ability to keep operating?
Demographic	Are there any human resource issues due to age, gender, distribution and number affecting the provision of services in your organization? Do you have an ageing workforce, or a workforce that is declining in numbers? Will patient care be dominated by the care of the elderly in future years, and will the health needs of women change as the trend towards more work and less children continues?
Sociological	What is the social class of your clients, and how does this impact on your service to them? What does an increasingly mobile population mean to the concept of community health care?
Economic	Has the trend from public to private ownership of national services impacted upon your organization, and what will happen in the future? Will the demands of fiscal accountability take precedence over quality of service? Will society invest more heavily in public or private health care in the future?

nurse practitioners; however, this may pose a threat to those practitioners who are not suitably qualified.

- *Technological*: web-based video cameras in patients' homes could dramatically alter the role of practitioners in outpatient clinics. Similarly, telemetry used to monitor patients' heart rhythms when they are at home could revolutionize the role of the coronary care unit, but these developments

and opportunities will only be available for those hospitals willing to invest in the information technology and communications infrastructure.

- *Demographic*: over the last decade there has been a reduction in the availability of qualified doctors in the UK. At the same time there has been a shortage of nurses. Some areas have been hit harder than others, making demographic considerations important when planning for the delivery of health care. In some cases this has led to opportunities for nurses to expand their role in the clinical setting with alternative models of skill mix in operation to deliver care in new ways. In other cases this has led to a restriction in nurses' development, with hospital management deciding that there are not enough nurses to do the work of nursing anyway, without allowing some of the workforce to expand their role and move away from the previous model of nursing. So you see how an analysis of the demographics could result in a conclusion that there is either an opportunity (the possibility of expanding the nurse's role) or a threat (a restriction on the movement of nurses beyond where they are at the present time).

The question of how to prioritize your external audit depends very much on whether you are trying to inform your own career decisions or preparing a departmental budget for a large hospital. If you regard an external audit as an ever-present radar that allows you to scan your external environment, then you are less likely to be caught by surprise as events beyond your immediate control impact on the delivery of your services to patients.

Internal audit

What you regard as your internal environment within the health care industry is not so easy to define. In the business world, this typically means the resources and capabilities of the company you are working for. However, in the case of a district nurse, for instance, is their 'company' the GP practice they are based in, the health authority they are employed by, or the district nursing team they work within? Because of the complexity of these working relationships, we have chosen to approach the completion of an internal audit by using a process akin to stakeholder mapping.

Kotler and Anderson (1996) use the concept of *publics* to determine who to include on any such stakeholder map and how to group them together. They define a public as:

... a distinct group of people, organizations, or both whose actual or potential needs must in some sense be served.

The four groups of publics relevant to our

stakeholder map – Input, Intermediary, Internal and Consuming publics – can be mapped as in Figure 10.2. We are defining each of these publics as follows:

- *Input* – a good way to think about Input publics is any person or group not directly owned or employed by your organization who can affect the delivery of your service to patients. We have broken them down into Donor, Supplier or Regulatory bodies, with several examples given in Figure 10.2 for the hospital setting.
- *Intermediary* – this describes either how you gain access to your patients (existing and potential) or how they gain access to you. In marketing terms, an intermediary will be involved in either a 'push' strategy (whereby you transmit information out through various channels in order to communicate with your patients) or a 'pull' strategy (whereby you have patients who are referred to you from a variety of sources). Examples of both are given in Figure 10.2.
- *Internal* – is just as it sounds, and who you might naturally think of as colleagues in the same organization that you work for.
- *Consuming* – is also a reasonably obvious group, comprising the people who use/receive the services you offer. In the case of nurse practitioner services it would be easy to assume that the users of the service are simply patients; however, consuming publics include the whole variety of people who could potentially walk through the hospital doors, such as family members, carers, GPs and others.

There are two important reasons to undertake this process:

1. If you consider your organization in isolation during your internal audit, then you will be missing the myriad of associated groups of people who affect the services you provide. For instance, in a hospital setting both cleaning and catering services are often outsourced, but you must consider them in your assessment of your organization's resources and capabilities (think what a patient's experience would be like if they went on strike).
2. This process also helps to portray how connected and interdependent certain groups of people are, and shows that you

may need to consider them differently in certain contexts. Local GPs, to take one example, may well be referring patients to your ward (so they are an Intermediary public) at the same time as they are working at your hospital as A&E cover (so they become an Internal public) while also needing to attend outpatients appointments as a patient (as a Consuming public). The

same GP might also end up on the Trust Board of the hospital as an Input public.

Do not forget, as you start to create your own stakeholder map, that you also have to consider each public that you list in terms of their strengths and weaknesses. This process will then inform both your vision and mission, and the formation of your strategic objectives

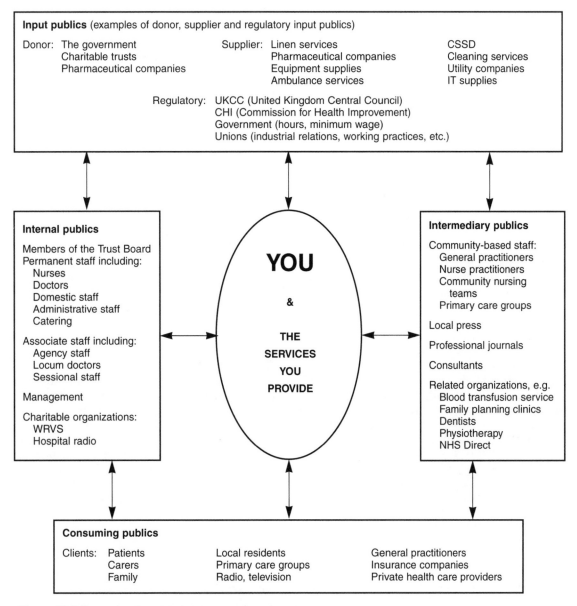

Figure 10.2 Example of a stakeholder map for a hospital setting.

in which you will endeavour to address the weaknesses and support the strengths.

Once you have completed your own version of this map, then it is time to make the transition from gathering data and ideas to turning them into a compelling vision for the future, along with a road map showing how to get there.

Vision and mission

Visions guide the best missions. A vision is a contagious dream.
(Kotler *et al.*, 1996)

A vision should paint 'an ideal and unique image of the future ... a target that beckons'.
(Zeithaml and Bitner, 1996)

Any visit to a business library will reveal an abundance of literature and a variety of quotes that are all trying to define what a vision should or shouldn't be. We are particularly fond of the two given above, simply because they encourage you to think beyond the immediate constraints of your daily routine and to imagine a situation that is markedly better than what presently exists for both your patients and yourself.

Given that visions should be something of an aspirational picture that everyone can remember, it is important to make sure that your mission articulates the purpose of your practice or organization. Missions are not something that should change every month; rather they need to connect the priorities of today with the vision of tomorrow in a way that is accessible to all relevant parties.

The mission should be a realistic, concise, distinct and motivating statement relating to the purpose of your service offering. A vision statement for an orthopaedic pre-operative assessment unit might well be along the lines of 'to become nationally renowned for the quality of our service to patients'. The mission statement that followed on from such a vision could be 'to offer solace, understanding and education to patients who have been listed for orthopaedic surgery by providing a safe, timely and accurate pre-operative assessment service'.

Neither the vision nor the mission should be considered independently from the research and analysis undertaken during the external and internal audits. The reason for this is so that you can understand the *context* in which your hospital or practice is operating, as well as the *priorities* for taking your organization/practice area forward.

Given that the vision and mission are concerned with *where* you want to go, we will now move on to thinking through *what* you are going to concentrate on in order get there, by creating a number of goals that will enable you to achieve that *contagious dream*.

Strategic objectives

Strategic objectives are your important goals. They will also provide the headings under which your more detailed plans (covered in the following section) are spelt out. In marketing terms, these goals are informed by the STP process, which is a simple amalgam of:

- Segmentation – identifying a group of users with common needs or characteristics
- Targeting – focusing your marketing mix to address a specific market segment
- Positioning – your place in the industry relative to other providers according to various criteria such as friendliness, professionalism, hygiene, access, efficiency, cost, etc., as perceived and defined by the patient.

Each strategic objective, therefore, should be clear in relation to whom it is aimed (i.e. segmentation), how it is going to address that segment (i.e. targeting) and how that group of patients regards your service (i.e. positioning). Let us look at each one of these factors in turn.

Segmentation
To borrow a turn of phrase from a number of politicians, the key to effective marketing is segmentation, segmentation, segmentation. What this is trying to illustrate is the importance of not generalizing about the people you serve or making the mistake of considering them to be all the same (you know you have been in nursing too long when you become convinced that the whole world is sick!). There is no single correct way of segmenting your patients; in fact, the more criteria you have to segment them by, the better equipped you will be to understand their needs and behaviour.

How would you group your patients according to their needs and characteristics? We tried to brainstorm the answer to this question from the perspective of a minor injuries unit in a hospital, and came up with the following list of questions:

1. Is it an injury or an illness?
2. Is it chronic or is it acute?
3. Is this person a child, an adult or an elderly person?
4. Are they alone or with friends/family?
5. Are they agitated or calm?
6. Do they comprehend your language/accent or not?
7. What is their gender, ethnicity, social class, occupation, age, sexual orientation, religion, and physical ability?
8. Are they likely to require your services again (how do you arrange follow-up)?
9. Do they require any medications?
10. Do they require any interventions from Social Services on discharge?
11. Can they afford the treatment that you are recommending?
12. Is travel to and from their home an issue?

and so on. ...

Naturally, if you pursued this process too far then you could define a market segment for every single patient and end up with a somewhat fragmented marketing strategy. Having spent some time thinking about your patients as members of different market segments, the next step is to determine which of these criteria are the most important in terms of meeting the needs of your patients.

Targeting

Which leads us on to targeting. If you were an accident and emergency nurse practitioner concerned about the growing number of teenage girls requesting emergency contraception from your unit, then you might well decide to target this group with a series of educational presentations in their schools/clubs/etc. through an alliance with a local family planning clinic. This would be an example of a targeted marketing campaign to serve the needs of a specific patient population.

Positioning

Staying with this example also helps to explain the concept of 'positioning', given that it is likely that you will only be successful in reaching this patient group if they are prepared to listen to what you have to say and change their behaviour accordingly. This has a lot to do with their perception of your hospital (compared with other health services that could provide them with emergency contraception) and how they regard you personally. Your perception of what comprises an effective service for this population could include clinically correct advice and timely prescribing. What they may regard as important, however, is whether or not you tell their parent(s) and how judgemental you are in relation to their lifestyle choices as young adults. The key to effective positioning is to understand how your patients regard the services you provide.

A well-written strategic objective will therefore be clear about the patient group you have identified (S) and it will cover how to approach that target group (T), bearing in mind *their* perspective of the services you provide (P). The STP process in a nutshell.

Flexible planning

In order to achieve any one of your strategic objectives, it will be necessary to develop a plan. One method of structuring your plan can be the use of a format called the 'marketing mix' or the seven 'P's. The seven 'P's include the product, price, place, promotion, people, processes and physical environment, and we will discuss each in turn.

The product

Defining the product in the health care setting is not always as easy as it might be if you were selling a packet of cornflakes. If your objective is to provide a high-quality and cost-effective nurse practitioner service to patients who attend the accident and emergency setting with minor injuries and illnesses, then the product can be seen as the total package of care experienced by patients attending the unit. The concept of a 'service offering' is therefore a more appropriate term for nursing. This might include issues regarding the patient's experience of the service, such as accessibility, waiting times, clarity of health education provided by the nurse practitioners, and provision of support on discharge from the service. The service offering might also include accessibility to important resources, such as the availability of radiology and the nurse practitioner's ability to refer for X-rays. A further important issue might be the availability of medications and the nurse practitioner's ability to provide patients with these medications. In the example of the nurse practitioner-led minor injuries unit the product can be seen as the service that the nurse practitioner provides, and clearly this includes the skills of the nurse; however, it also includes other elements of the service, such as access to support services and the workload of the staff. An example of the action required when considering this service offering would therefore include ensuring that the nurse practitioners had access to radiology and could administer medications according to patient group directions, that there were enough staff to minimize the waiting time of the patients, and that the nurse practitioners were educated to provide a holistic, safe and effective service.

The price

When related to health care in the UK, the 'price' can be interpreted as the value to the patient of the service offering versus the cost of delivering that service. It is often difficult to determine the economics of the service; however, value can be assessed by focusing on the patient's experience. An example of this might be a rheumatology nurse practitioner who has been consulting with patients in the outpatient setting. The strategic objective might be to provide an accessible nurse practitioner service for patients with rheumatoid arthritis, which might include outreach clinics in the community setting. The value for the patients could be measured in terms of their satisfaction with the service and their comments on the provision of a service closer to home. It might also include the patients' experience of consulting with a nurse practitioner as opposed to a senior house officer in a busy outpatients setting. We could anticipate that the patients would be less stressed in the community setting than they might be in the hospital environment; they may be educated more effectively by the nurse practitioner, who has the skill to communicate health-promoting messages to the patient; and they may feel more able to share their feelings with the nurse than when they are acutely aware of the pressures of time in the outpatients setting. It is important then to consider the meaning of the word 'price' or 'value' when planning the necessary interventions to achieve your strategic objectives, and to put in place the structures that will enable your service to achieve that value. Obviously this has to be considered within the strictures of cost effectiveness over the longer term. In the example provided above, the action required might include investing in the knowledge and skills of the nurse practitioner to ensure that the service provided is safe and effective.

The place

In marketing terms, this often relates to the distribution channels used to get your products to market. Translated into nursing, this involves the activities that surround the delivery of health services to your patients. You need to consider how and where you make your service offering available. Nurse practitioners are increasingly working on the boundaries of primary and secondary care. Services that were once seen as the domain of the hospital setting are now being provided in the community. In addition to the physical location, you might also need to consider *how* the service is provided. With developments in information technology there are many models of alternative provision of services depending upon the specific needs of the local population. Dermatology services can be provided by telemedicine links to GP surgeries, advice on minor injuries and illnesses can be provided over the telephone by the NHS Direct triage system, and video-conferencing can allow a consultant in a hospital setting to talk with a patient who is many miles away in an inaccessible rural location. In the example of a dermatology nurse practitioner, then, the services can be made available in an outpatients clinic, in a community clinic and via telemedicine. In planning the activities required to meet the strategic objective of providing a nurse practitioner dermatology service to the local population, it would be important to consider investing in the necessary information technology to provide telemedicine and to negotiate with the health care team in the community setting to provide a suitable clinic for the provision of the outreach service.

Promotion

This involves publicity and the methods you use to inform your target population of the services you plan to provide. It is clearly important to communicate effectively with the intended clientele to explain the service and highlight its merits. There is clearly a problem with a poster that advertises a nurse practitioner walk-in centre with a picture of a nurse examining a baby, when the service is only available to children aged 2 years and above (Lipman, 2000). The promotional materials need to be directed to the target audience and realistically reflect the service provided. In some areas this may mean developing promotional leaflets that are written in several languages to ensure that the local population understand what the service is about. It may be possible to use local newspapers, radio and television to highlight the developments that are taking place in your hospital setting. It is also important to consider the promotion that takes place when the patient accesses the service. Posters and videos in waiting rooms, well-versed reception staff and the use of leaflets distributed in the clinical area can help to reinforce the message and promote the services offered.

These publicity activities are typical of what is known as a 'push' strategy, whereby information is pushed out towards your intended patient group through various channels. Another way to approach promotion is the 'pull' strategy, whereby patients are referred to your practice or clinic through various intermediaries (see Figure 10.2 for examples). If patients are being referred to you inappropriately, then it becomes your responsibility to educate your intermediaries (i.e. promote awareness).

People

It is important to consider *all* of the people involved in the provision of the service you are trying to market, and to ensure that they are sufficiently skilled to carry out their respective roles. The focus may be a nurse practitioner-led heart failure clinic based in the hospital outpatients setting. The tendency in this situation would be to ensure that the nurse practitioners were adequately educated and prepared for their role. It is clearly important, however, to ensure that the reception staff are prepared for their role in directing patients to the service, that support staff are prepared for their role in carrying out venepuncture electrocardiograms and other investigations, and that the consultants know when it is appropriate to make a referral to the nurse practitioner clinic. The action necessary to achieve the strategic objective might be to provide a period of

training for the staff and put in place some structured clinical supervision to develop their skills.

Processes

There are a number of processes in operation that will have an impact upon a strategic objective. An example of a process might be the methods that nurse practitioners use to arrange for patients to receive the medications they need. The process might be that they arrange for a prescription to be generated by a doctor and then hand this to the patient, who goes off to the pharmacy to collect their medication. Alternatively, the nurse practitioners might be using patient care directions to guide their decisions about medications. In this instance, a different process would be in place where the nurses assess the patient, apply the presenting situation to the patient care direction and then make a decision about the medication. The medication would then be supplied to the patient in the department. You can see therefore that a service that utilizes the process of doctor-signed prescriptions would be different and arguably less efficient than a service that uses patient care directions. This particular example does however highlight the need to consider all the Ps in planning the activities to achieve your strategic objectives, as the use of patient care directions in the absence of adequately educated nurse practitioners could be seen as potentially unsafe for patients. Other processes that could be considered include referral patterns between nurse practitioners and consultants, between GPs and nurse practitioners, or the process of ordering X-rays from the radiology department.

Physical environment

Clearly this refers to the physical setting where the service is delivered, and is also referred to as physical evidence. Physical evidence includes the way in which you promote your physical environment on leaflets or brochures. The environment needs to be welcoming and comfortable. Consider the nurse practitioner operating out of an office at the end of a corridor with seating lined up outside the door for the waiting patients. A situation such as this conveys a message to patients about the value of the service they are receiving. Consider also the amount of noise in the area, the appearance of the room and even the size of the room. It is helpful to think of the physical environment from the patients' and carers' perspective, and therefore it may be useful to enlist their help in assessing the surroundings of the clinic by using patient questionnaires or interviews.

Having used the structure of the seven Ps to identify the activities you might engage in to achieve your strategic objectives, you will have developed a marketing plan. You have thought about a wide range of issues that impact upon the service, and have considered approaches to market your service more effectively. The next stage is to move on and actually put this plan into action.

Implementation

If you are a single nurse practitioner trying to promote the service you provide, you will need to organize your job so that you are able to implement the marketing plan in your day-to-day practice. You may need to liaise with others who have access to the resources you require to implement your plan, or you may need to identify time in your working week to devote to the various activities you need to engage in.

If you are responsible for the work of others, you may need to consider the function of other people's jobs and organize them appropriately. This may involve altering job descriptions and developing the team to ensure that everyone is engaged in the process. It will be necessary to develop performance targets and to provide feedback to your staff team on an ongoing basis and during regular appraisals. One pitfall to avoid in developing this process is to end up with a 'shopping list' of targets for your staff to achieve. Time must be taken to prioritize your ambitions so that everyone is clear as to the most important developments that need to take place. Many businesses will use the term Key Performance Indicators (KPIs) to highlight this point.

The implementation stage is basically getting the job done, and the way in which you approach this will depend upon the service you are trying to market and the plan you have developed during your marketing analysis.

Monitoring and evaluation

Once you have implemented your plan it is crucial to monitor and evaluate the process,

particularly in relation to your Key Performance Indicators. The success of the implementation of your marketing plan can be assessed using a variety of measures, including clinical audit, patient satisfaction questionnaires, interviews and outcome measures (such as prescribing data and numbers of people using your service). Your service might also be monitored externally by an organization such as the Commission for Health Improvement (CHI), who aim to promote high-quality health care services by independently scrutinizing local clinical governance arrangements (DoH, 2000b). An organization such as the CHI can provide the benchmarks for you to measure your own service against. It can also identify examples of best practice, which might help you to critique your service.

Monitoring and evaluating the implementation of your marketing plan will provide information that can be used to improve your marketing strategy even further. The results can have an impact on your vision, may alter your strategic objectives, influence your flexible planning or change the way in which you implement your plan. The whole system is a dynamic, flexible approach to the evaluation and promotion of the services you offer, and as such it can help you to cope more effectively with the pressures on your role, your work, your ward or your department.

Conclusion

This chapter has explored the use of marketing with particular reference to the role of the nurse practitioner. We have provided you with a framework for thinking about marketing in your setting, which has broadly addressed methods of gathering information and ideas, transferring this information into strategic objectives and breaking these down further into specific plans which are then followed by a process of review and evaluation. All of this takes place under the umbrella of relationship marketing, which places a clear emphasis on the importance of your interactions with all the people identified on the stakeholder map.

Marketing is both a set of activities and a way of thinking that can and should enrich your service offering. Ultimately we hope that by following the flowchart in Figure 10.1 you will be better able to meet the needs of your patients and enable nurse practitioners to implement their roles in clinical practice more effectively.

References

Brownlie, D. (1988). Analysing the environment. In: *Marketing Handbook*, 3rd edn (M. J. Thomas, ed.). Gower Publishing, Hants, UK, pp. 20–46.

Chartered Institute of Marketing (2000). Information and Library Services. http://www.-cim.co.uk

Department of Health (2000a). http://www.doh.gov.uk/nurseprescribing

Department of Health (2000b). Commission for Health Improvement. http://www.doh.gov.uk/chi/index.htm

HMSO (1968). *Medicines Act*. HMSO.

Kotler, P. and Anderson, A. R. (1996). *Strategic Marketing for Nonprofits Organizations*. Prentice-Hall.

Kotler, P., Armstrong, G., Saunders, J. and Wong, V. (1996). *Principles of Marketing*. Prentice-Hall.

Lipman, T. (2000). The secret life of the NHS. *Br. Med. J.*, **321,** 894.

McDermott, B. (1996). Marketing nursing. *Nursing Standard*, **10(20),** 49–52.

Watts, G. (1996). Marketing planning, implementation and control. Lecture notes, Lancaster University Marketing Management programme.

Young A. P. (1995). Is marketing an obligatory skill in the nursing role? *Br. J. Nursing*, **4(6),** 965–8.

Zeithaml, V. A. and Bitner, M. J. (1996). *Services Marketing*, McGraw-Hill. Singapore.

11

EVALUATING THE NURSE PRACTITIONER ROLE IN HOSPITAL

Mike Walsh and Shirley Reveley

The first blossom was the best blossom
For the child who had never seen an orchard.
From *Apple Blossom*, by Louis MacNeice (1982)

Introduction

As Louis MacNeice observes in the above quotation, first impressions count for a great deal, but they can be very misleading. A key element in developing the nurse practitioner role is rigorous evaluation to discover how well the role is working (and why) and to investigate problem areas in order that remedial action may be taken. Superficial first impressions are not acceptable as evidence upon which to base practice. MacNeice's words also have another message for us, as however beautiful apple blossom may be, it is only the beginning of a longer story. If the apple tree is properly looked after and nurtured, it will subsequently yield fruit that is even more useful than blossom. So it is with the nurse practitioner; a successful start to a service is encouraging, but properly supported it can lead on to many subsequent benefits that may not have been apparent in the early days. Put another way, if a hospital wants to reap the full benefits of a nurse practitioner service, it has to be seen as a medium- to long-term investment that needs looking after and supporting, just like an orchard does!

This chapter will contain a brief overview of some of the key points involved in evaluating the nurse practitioner role in hospital settings. This should assist the nurse involved in developing a new nurse practitioner service to ensure that it is properly evaluated and also critically to review published research looking at the nurse practitioner role. Evaluation is essential for several reasons, not least of which is the need for rapid feedback concerning the effectiveness and quality of the service provided.

The clinical governance agenda means that nurse practitioner services have to achieve clinical effectiveness. This means that an intervention such as a nurse practitioner service ideally has to be able to show that it will '... do what it is intended to do i.e. maintain and improve health and secure the greatest possible health gain' (DoH, 1996). A. Kitson (First National Conference on Evidence-Based Nursing, London, February 1997, Unpublished) provided a simple shorthand version of this definition of clinical effectiveness when she defined it as doing the right things, and doing things right. The evidence-based practice movement that came to the fore in the late 1990s means that we have to have evidence to support what we are doing. Any nurse practitioner service therefore needs to gather evidence of its effectiveness, whilst publication of such evidence informs and assists others to develop their services elsewhere. Opposition to the nurse practitioner concept can only be overcome by producing evidence of its effectiveness, whilst hospital Trust managers will not support nurse practitioner innovations unless evidence is provided as part of the marketing strategy. Evaluation and evidence are therefore as essential as education in setting up nurse practitioner services.

Collecting the evidence

The reputed last words of Gertrude Stein were, 'What is the answer? ... In that case, What is the question?' (Sutherland, 1951). As it is with deathbed speeches so it is with research, as the key to good research is to ask the right questions to begin with! To evaluate a nurse practitioner service we therefore have to start off with the right questions, which should be related to the goals of the service that is being provided. Only if you know what you are trying to achieve can you find out whether you have achieved it. There are probably three broad types of research question that could be asked:

1. Is the nurse practitioner service as good as/better than the existing service? (assuming that one exists). This usually involves comparison with an existing medically-led service. A range of criteria will be used to measure how the services compare, such as patient satisfaction, clinical outcomes or cost effectiveness.
2. How does the nurse practitioner service impact upon patients? This question is likely to be asked where a completely new service is being set up, as well as where a comparison with existing services is being made.
3. What is the impact of the nurse practitioner service elsewhere in the National Health Service?

Nursing research has traditionally been biased towards a qualitative approach, whilst medicine has tended to travel down the quantitative road. This is not the place for a lengthy discussion about these two research paradigms and their relative merits. Put simply, qualitative research seeks to describe the way the world is and how it appears to people taking part in events. It therefore relies heavily upon words as the raw units of data, and does not deal in hypotheses and statistics. Quantitative research, on the other hand, is about setting up hypotheses and testing them by gathering statistical data or using numerical information derived from surveys to describe what is happening in the real world. Both methods have their strengths and weaknesses, and each is appropriate in some situations but not others. A very simplified explanation might be to say that quantitative research will tell you what is happening, but to find out why people behave the way they do you need a qualitative approach because that is the only way you will obtain their point of view. Of course it is much more complicated than this in many situations, but hopefully this simplified account will help the reader who has not done a research methods course to understand the basic differences between these two main research methods.

The first type of question listed above needs a quantitative approach to obtain a clear answer, although qualitative data would also be valuable. The qualitative paradigm comes to the fore in dealing with the second type of question, whilst the third question needs an approximately equal mix of approaches.

A further term needs to be introduced here, *action research*. This relatively new approach to research is concerned with rapid feedback from data gathered in the field, which permits modification of a project while it is still ongoing. The project can therefore evolve and change in response to continual evaluation. The traditional alternative is to set up a research protocol or design, run the project consistently in a set way, and gather data, which is used to finally pass judgement on whether a project succeeded or not. The data could also be used to test a hypothesis, which can be pronounced confirmed or refuted at the end of the study.

Setting up a nurse practitioner service is a multidisciplinary exercise, and evaluation should reflect this multidisciplinary nature by drawing on both the quantitative and qualitative research traditions. Medical colleagues may need persuading about the value of including qualitative data, but quantitative data alone will never tell the full story. It is of course essential to know objective details, such as how many patients the nurse practitioner saw, what percentage were treated in accordance with agreed guidelines, and percentage scores of patient satisfaction. But it is also essential to know what the patient thought about their nurse practitioner consultation, the opinions of doctors and other nurses about the new service, and how things appear to the nurse practitioner as she reflects upon progress of the project. Nurses may also need persuading that gathering objective statistical data is a necessary part of evaluation. However, this is the language that medicine and senior NHS managers understand. Nurse practitioner services require a true spirit of multidisciplinary co-operation, and this extends to a mutual respect for the different research traditions of the groups involved. Good evaluation explores both quantitative and qualitative perspectives in order to obtain a rounded view of the real world.

The key principles of action research make it a valuable tool for developing new and innovative services, although medicine may not be very familiar with action research as a methodology. We have already argued that a new nurse practitioner service should have a project team to develop the service and oversee it for the first year or two until it is firmly bedded down. The project team must have the nurse practitioner(s) as full members. The action research approach leads to data being gathered as the project proceeds, and this can be fed into regular meetings of the project team for action. Problems become apparent as they arise and can be dealt with promptly as a result of discussion amongst the team members, leading to decisions to change practice which are timely and supported by the project team. The nurse practitioner involved in delivering the service is pivotal to this process, and therefore is a key member of the project team.

In any evaluation study it is necessary to determine at the outset who will be gathering the data. There are some types of data where only the nurse practitioner can gather the information, and there are other types where the nurse practitioner should actually be the last person to gather data. A reflective diary kept by the nurse practitioner as part of the project can be a rich source of personal perspectives on progress. Only the nurse practitioner can produce this kind of information, and the actual diary itself should be confidential to the nurse practitioner. However, it can provide a source for the nurse practitioner to provide summaries about feelings and ideas for the project team that can be incorporated in the final evaluation report.

The need for patient confidentiality means that it is often best if the nurse practitioner gathers summary data concerning presenting conditions and treatment. Audit of performance standards should either be carried out by another person or, if the nurse practitioner audits his or her own work, there should be an anonymized sample that is checked by a second person. This is essential to deal with any accusations of bias.

Patient interviews about the service should be carried out by a neutral third person who is skilled in research. This will ensure that bias does not creep into patient accounts, either because the patient does not wish to appear critical of the nurse practitioner or because the nurse practitioner may (possibly unconsciously) influence what the patient says. It certainly deals with the suspicion that the nurse practitioner may have edited or selectively quoted the patient comments in order to appear in the best light.

Evaluation of a nurse practitioner service therefore requires the use of both quantitative and qualitative methods and should ideally be multidisciplinary in nature, incorporating an action research methodology. An outside body such as a local university nursing department should be involved in the research process in order that appropriate research expertise be brought to bear on the problem. This also protects the evaluation from charges of bias, as neutral third parties will be involved in data gathering and analysis.

If nursing developments are to be evaluated, this must be done rigorously. The gold standard for evidence is the randomized controlled trial (RCT), and an evaluation that uses an RCT methodology will provide the strongest evidence of cause and effect. This assumes that there is a comparison being made between the new nurse practitioner service and the existing service, of course. In this case, patients should be allocated at random to either the nurse practitioner or the existing service and their treatment consistently delivered by one or the other route. The results of treatment should be measured using the same standard measuring tool by a neutral researcher. In order to demonstrate any differences and minimize possible bias due to a small sample, a large sample of patients is required. Polit and Hungler (1995) offer a detailed discussion of power analysis, which is an essential concept in determining the size of the sample that would be expected to show a statistically significant difference if such a difference existed. The study by Sakr *et al.* (1999) comparing the performance of nurse practitioners and junior doctors is a good example of an RCT that illustrates these points.

The RCT approach does not sit easily with the action research methodology discussed earlier, however, as the continual feedback and adjustments involved in action research are at odds with the control element of an RCT. It is also possible that the type of client group being worked with is not suitable for an RCT methodology, such as the outreach nurse practitioner service for female sex workers described by Hunter (2000). Whilst the RCT provides powerful evidence it simply may not be appropriate for some situations, and the more flexible action research methodology will be better suited in those cases. By the same token, the kind of data being gathered has to be tailored to the nature of the project. The example cited above of a nurse practitioner service for female sex workers can gather some objective data, such as number of women seen by the nurse practitioner. However, qualitative data on a case study basis about the difference the service makes to the women's lives is the key evidence that can be used to make a valid judgement on the service. The type of data gathered is of course determined by the goal of the service and the research question being asked.

Evaluation of a service can only take place effectively if there is clear agreement on what the service is to achieve (service level provision). Chapter 1 stressed the need for clear and agreed project goals in setting up the nurse practitioner service. Apart from this being important from a change management perspective it is crucial for evaluation, as this tells the researchers, and ultimately the project team, where the goalposts are. Knowing the projected outcomes of the project ensures that the researchers gather the correct data and allows the project team to then use that data to judge whether the service is succeeding. If success is to be measured in terms of effective change, then it is essential that baseline data are gathered prior to setting up the nurse practitioner service. Knowing the goal of the service ensures that the correct baseline data are gathered.

In the example of female sex workers discussed above, the goal is to improve their access to health care. Baseline data about their existing health practices needs to be gathered and, by the nature of the lifestyle involved, this may involve the researcher working indirectly through the nurse practitioner, who has the one-to-one contact necessary to build up a picture of each woman's individual health problems. Gaining access to and the confidence of the women in order that a third person may evaluate the service may prove difficult and even impossible, in which case the researcher acts as a resource for the nurse practitioner to carry out the actual evaluation. This means that the nurse practitioner actually obtains the research data as the clients talk about how the service has affected them. The researcher assists in the interpretation, analysis and validation of the raw data that the nurse practitioner obtains. Evaluation would look at

the impact that the woman feels the nurse practitioner service has had on her life, which is an example of the second type of question posed on page 131.

Consider a more conventional example next: comparing a new nurse practitioner service with an existing service. A pre-operative nurse practitioner-led assessment project may be set up with the goal of reducing the number of cancelled operations. Anecdotal evidence may suggest that cancellations are due to patients being unfit for anaesthesia or simply not turning up on the day of their surgery. As the researcher knows the goal of the study is to reduce cancellations, the first thing to do is to establish a baseline against which to measure. The researcher therefore checks back through existing data to work out the number of cancellations in the last year and looks for any patterns such as the effects of the time of year. With baseline data secure, the researcher can monitor cancellation rates once the nurse practitioner service is up and running and a simple answer to the question of whether the service is effective may be found. However, it might also be possible for the researcher to work with the nurse practitioner to investigate why patients did not attend for surgery or why they were declared unfit. This information informs nurse practitioner practice (action research) and can lead to strategies to deal with particular recurring themes, such as chronic medical problems like diabetes not being dealt with before surgery. Assessment could lead to a simple step, such as bringing diabetic patients into hospital a day before surgery in order to stabilize them on a sliding scale insulin and intravenous fluid regimen. Knowing the goal of the project ensures that the right questions are asked and the right data gathered to answer the key research questions involving the clinical effectiveness of the new service.

Another approach may be to run an RCT in which existing conventional services operate alongside the new nurse practitioner service, and the two are compared after an agreed period of time or number of patients. This presents the logistical problem of running two different services together and in such a way that one does not interfere with the other. The practical difficulties of this may lead to a different approach, known as a time series design, in which the nurse practitioner service becomes fully operational, replacing the medical service, and runs for an agreed period of time. The results of the service are then compared with previous performance before the nurse practitioner began work. For this to be a valid comparison there have to be no other major changes that have occurred at the same time that may explain any observed differences in performance, such as medical staffing problems or moving to a new hospital. If all other circumstances are known to be the same, it is likely that any observed difference is due to the introduction of the nurse practitioner. It is not possible to say, however, that any improvement is definitely due to the nurse practitioner, as there may be other factors at work that are unknown to the researcher and clinical staff. Herein lies the weakness of the time series design as opposed to the RCT, as the control element of the RCT greatly reduces the chances of other unforeseen factors producing the effects that are observed.

An alternative example might involve setting up a nurse practitioner-run outpatients service to manage patients with urological problems. The key question is again, what is the objective of the service? It might be to improve the quality of life enjoyed by patients, but it may be to provide closer monitoring of disease progress by having more frequent appointments. These are two different objectives requiring different kinds of data to be gathered. The 'quality of life' goal requires baseline assessment of the quality of life enjoyed by patients, utilizing interview or questionnaire techniques, under the existing system. The same data then need to be collected after the nurse practitioner service has been implemented. If monitoring disease progress is the goal, the researcher must look at different types of data relating to mortality and morbidity statistics, which must again be gathered as a baseline before implementing the new service and afterwards. Whichever of these two questions is being asked, it would be possible to set up an RCT or a time series design as outlined in the preceding paragraph.

Obviously, the goal of the service will have major implications for the service provided by the nurse practitioner. In the quality of life scenario, the nurse practitioner will be exploring holistically how the person is coping and offering a mix of practical advice, patient teaching and supportive therapies using his or her assessment skills. In the disease-monitoring scenario, the emphasis will be more on screening and investigations. A clear goal at the outset will ensure that the nurse practitioner knows where he or she is going, and the researcher gathers the correct data to answer the question of whether or not the service is effective. It is easy, however, to see how the quality of life and disease-monitoring goals could become muddled, leading to confusion with different professional perspectives leading to different priorities. Clear goal statements at the beginning should avoid this problem.

Evaluation research

Evaluation research is closely linked to action research, and is becoming more widely used nowadays. It provides an alternative to the positivist research paradigm, and recognizes that real life is complex, unpredictable and often messy. Beattie (1984) and Smith and Cantley (1985) are proponents of evaluation research, and the following section offers a brief overview of their work. According to the World Health Organisation (1981):

Evaluation implies judgement based on careful assessment and critical appraisal of given situations, which should lead to drawing sensible conclusions and making useful proposals for future action.

This definition reflects 'traditional' evaluative research, which, according to Smith and Cantley (1985), is a linear process in which service goals are defined, outcomes as measures of goal attainment are specified, criteria for success are identified, the effects are isolated from other possible causes, achievements are measured and a judgement is made on the success or otherwise of the service (innovation). This process has been described above. Whilst Smith and Cantley admit that this is undoubtedly an oversimplification of traditional evaluative research, they maintain that there is a high degree of consensus amongst commentators that these are the main characteristics of mainstream evaluative research, and cite Illsley (1980), Bulmer (1982) and Goldberg and Connelly (1982) in support of their argument.

A major problem with the traditional mode of evaluation research is that it appears to be a straightforward endeavour but in practice can be very demanding, not least because of the unpredictability of the real-life situations that evaluative research tends to be involved in exploring. Smith and Cantley (1985) argue that a mode of evaluative research has come about which is essentially experimental, rationalist and objectivist. This, they suggest, is fraught with difficulty, because it rests on certain assumptions about social policy, social research and organizations which are unjustified. They term these the 'presumption of rationality in social policy, the presumption of the experimental ideal in social research and the presumption of consensus in organisations'.

Drawing on the work of Carley (1982), Smith and Cantley suggest that policy is conceived and implemented by 'rational man' through a series of linked activities as follows: a problem is identified and values organized, all solutions are listed, consequences are predicted, consequences are compared and a strategy is selected on the basis of costs and benefits. All is well with this process if the character of what is being evaluated and the method of evaluation 'fit'. However, the steps in the process described above are an ideal model, and a model is not reality. The rationalistic approach omits a variety of important political factors, not least of which is the power of vested interests (Smith and May, 1980). The rational model assumes that the goals of the organization are clearly articulated, and this too is not borne out in practice (Smith and Cantley, 1985, p. 5):

Ambiguity and confusion of purpose are typical and not at all unusual features of most agencies. A good deal of research in hospitals and other organisations has shown that objectives vary within and between significant groups. Goals of service are complex, multiple, conflicting and vary over time and between contexts. They are variously interpreted, notoriously ambiguous, and are sometimes difficult to locate at all.

The presumption of the experimental ideal leads to a perception that the experimental (the randomized control trial discussed above) or quasi-experimental design is the desirable mode of research as advocated by Richardson and Maynard (1995) when they state that:

The cost-effectiveness of substituting nurses for doctors cannot be demonstrated without the measurement of the quality of the services provided. ... To estimate the level at which doctors can be

substituted with nurses in the UK would require a randomized control trial with careful measurement of costs and patients' outcomes and an adequate follow-up period ... the costs of a properly controlled trial may be small when compared to the potential savings available by substituting nurses for doctors and the potential costs (including damage to patients) of changing skill mix 'on the hoof' and in the absence of a sufficient knowledge base. It is inefficient, but usual, for the NHS and other health care systems to alter skill mix and pay little regard to the evaluation of such policies.

However, in practice this is very difficult to undertake as there are ethical and practical constraints such as the problem of assigning patients or clients randomly to treatment and control groups. Also, researchers learn as they proceed, so there is usually instability in evaluative research. Participants can become aware of the different treatments, which also introduces bias. In any event, randomized control trials or experiments tell us what happened but rarely tell us why (Smith and Cantley, 1985).

The presumption of consensus within professional organizations is often made in evaluative research; an 'image of unity' which suggests that there is some objective or correct view of what is happening, the task of the researcher being to ascertain this objective truth (Smith and Cantley, 1985). These writers argue that frequently consensus does not exist, and researchers equate the interests of the institution as a whole with the interests of senior managers and officials. They argue for a more subjectivist methodology to promote the multiple perspectives within a given programme, which may not necessarily be in agreement with one another, and incorporate them into the evaluation. Thus ambiguity and lack of agreement between interest groups would become central to the research. This implies a need for an investigation of processes.

There is a range of stakeholders involved in the nurse practitioner initiative, each holding varying values and having unequal power. Each has invested different things and will be looking for different results. Managers, for example, will be looking for cost effectiveness. Doctors may want to know how the innovation benefits them and their patients, nursing staff will want to know how the role of the nurse practitioner impacts on themselves in relation to patients and colleagues, and nurse practitioners will want to know whether their way of working is acceptable. Patients may be concerned with issues of safety, accessibility and acceptability. Another stakeholder in process evaluation is the researcher, who has a stake in the project in terms of helping to make it work. There are also what Beattie (1984) describes as 'institutional agendas' to be considered. Here the evaluation is concerned with the identification and 'mapping' of the social, political and cultural context within which a particular programme is conducted, and attempting accurately to present its impact. This impact may relate to (Beattie, 1984, p. 6):

... the debates and conflicts to which a programme contributes in a particular agency or its particular professional groups; it may the discrepancy between a particular programme and wider prevailing climates. ...

The debates and conflicts surrounding the role of the nurse practitioner are receiving widespread attention in the nursing and medical press. The debate appears to be happening at different levels from the national nursing statutory body (United Kingdom Central Council for Nurses, Midwives and Health Visitors) through professional groups such as the Royal College of Nursing, the British Medical Association and educational institutions, who are trying to decide the kind and level of education and training nurse practitioners require. Conflicts surround the level at which the nurse practitioner practises (specialist or advanced practitioner), and how the role relates to other nursing roles such as that of the clinical nurse specialist. Conflict also relates to the use of the title 'nurse practitioner' – whether this is appropriate, whether it has 'elitist' connotations, and indeed the fact that all nurses are 'practitioners'. There is conflict regarding role boundaries within the nursing profession, and also role boundaries between the nursing and medical profession with which it has become closely allied.

Beattie (1984) suggests that the type of evaluation project he describes often takes the form of a case study and ends in a 'portrayal of the natural history of a particular intervention programme'. It tells the story of how the intervention runs its course, what kinds of thing support or obstruct it, what interests are brought to bear on it and how success and failure are decided and by whom. Pluralistic evaluation therefore utilizes data of whatever kind is able to address the issues of a range of stakeholders in the innovation. It involves the use of a range of methods. Beattie (1984, p. 8) calls this a 'multifaceted portfolio' approach, and suggests that it helps to overcome the limitations of using a 'unidimensional evaluation strategy':

Evaluation is a complex, elusive business, akin perhaps to a detective story, that requires all clues to be followed up that may lead to the understanding and resolution of a case in point. ...

One of the main objectives of evaluation research is to arrive at a decision as to whether an innovation has been successful. However, again this is no simple task as success means different things to different people. Smith and Cantley (1985) argue that success is measured differently by stakeholders according to whether their particular objectives are met. In this study success may be measured, depending on whose perspective is being taken into account, in terms of:

- Value for money (governments and managers)
- Easing pressure on doctors (health authorities and the medical profession)
- Offering an alternative service to patients
- Providing a quality service (health service policy makers, medical practitioners, health authorities)
- Increasing the rate of patient flow and patient satisfaction (managers)
- Public safety and the successful integration of a new nursing role into nursing practice (some elements of the nursing profession).

Reveley (1999) used this methodology to evaluate the introduction of a triage nurse practitioner into a group general practice.

Structuring the evidence

It may be a daunting prospect to look at a new nurse practitioner project and wonder where to begin in collecting evidence that will demonstrate how effective the service has become. There is however a useful framework which originates in the field of quality assurance and has been proposed by Øvetreit (1992). He considers that health service quality can be considered from the perspectives of professional, managerial and consumer quality. A new nurse practitioner service can therefore be evaluated by investigating:

- Professional quality, by measuring the achievement of clinical standards
- Managerial quality, by measuring the cost effectiveness of the service
- Consumer quality, by exploring patient satisfaction.

Professional quality

There has always been understandable concern that clinical mistakes may occur as the nurse practitioner begins to tread on traditional medical turf by seeing patients as the first point of contact and enjoying high levels of autonomy in management. This has led to a tendency to compare the performance of the nurse practitioner with that of a doctor as evidence of clinical quality. Such an approach tends to focus heavily on outcomes rather than the process of care. The recognition that the law would require a nurse practitioner to demonstrate the same level of competence as a doctor when carrying out work that has traditionally been seen as medical is a strong argument behind this approach to evaluation. Patients would also expect the nurse practitioner to be as competent as the doctor if they were seeing the nurse practitioner instead of the doctor. Falling below previous medical standards would also represent a deterioration in service provision and would be unacceptable.

All of the above statements are, of course, true; however, the situation is not quite so clear-cut, as certain implicit assumptions have been made. The above analysis assumes that the nurse practitioner is a straight substitute for a doctor and provides a medical consultation. In reality, the nurse is using medical (and nursing) skills to provide a nurse practitioner consultation. The use of medical skills means that the legal point raised above is of course perfectly valid, so for example the nurse practitioner would have to be as competent as the doctor in listening to breath sounds or carrying out a neurological examination. However, the process of the consultation may be very different to that which

occurs with a doctor. Evaluation should look at the nature of the consultation as well as the outcome, especially as the research question may shift from 'Are nurse practitioner consultations successful?' to 'Why are nurse practitioner consultations so successful?'.

The evaluation strategy should therefore avoid the trap of seeking a direct comparison between nurse practitioner and doctor, as there are significant differences in the nature of the consultation. There is a further assumption here, which is that the medical consultation provides the gold standard against which all else is compared. Doctors can, however, make mistakes, particularly more junior doctors. A clinical error rate of 10 per cent in junior hospital doctors seeing minor injuries has been found (p. 97), whilst in some circumstances nurse practitioners can outperform junior doctors in terms of ordering and interpreting radiographs. If a trial is to be made of nurse practitioners' clinical performance, then senior doctors should decide whether practice has met agreed criteria, rather than juniors who may make clinically significant errors themselves.

Above all, the nurse practitioner consultation is intrinsically different to a medical consultation, unless the role has actually been set up purely as one of medical substitution providing only a medical service such as preoperative clerking. In this case, however, the nurse is arguably not working as a nurse practitioner but rather as a physician's assistant if she has no authority or autonomy to act on her findings. The fact that a nurse practitioner consultation may take longer than a medical consultation is again not of importance if the different nature of the consultation is considered. The chances are that the more holistic approach of the nurse practitioner will result in time saved later.

Managerial quality

This is concerned with the cost-effective use of resources, and follows on from the previous discussion concerning direct comparisons with medicine. It is simple to add up the cost of a nurse practitioner and a doctor, divide by the number of patients seen and decide the relative cost per patient. However, this only gives a superficial view of whether the nurse practitioner service is cost effective relative to medicine, and there are many other factors to be taken into account.

Training costs must be considered. A nurse practitioner, once trained, is likely to stay in a role for a period of several years, whereas junior doctors rotate every 6 months and need retraining. A significant amount of that training is provided by experienced nursing staff. The inexperience of junior doctors means that they are, initially at least, likely to be slower in seeing patients and more prone to make mistakes or order unnecessary investigations. Factors such as these need to be costed into any comparisons. The same considerations also apply to evaluating the performance of a nurse practitioner, who is likely to be performing at a higher standard with the benefit of a year's experience in role than after only a few weeks.

The fact that a nurse practitioner consultation is different from a medical consultation also has to be considered in making cost comparisons. The nurse practitioner consultation may include a significant amount of patient education, use of counselling skills and exploration of family and emotional problems, all of which have a direct bearing on eventual outcomes. This does take time and could therefore make nurse practitioner consultations more expensive, even though in the long run they may represent better value for money. The nurse practitioner may also carry out certain nursing procedures that in a medical consultation might be delegated to other nurses, allowing the doctor to move on and see another patient more quickly. Elements such as these have to be factored into calculations about cost.

Unfortunately, many of the benefits of nurse practitioner consultations are not easily quantified in cost terms because they tend to prevent things happening later, after the consultation. If the evaluation is restricted to a simple comparison of doctors and nurse practitioners based on the cost of patients seen per hour, it will miss the benefits that accrue in the days and weeks after the consultation. To be a valid study it should try to measure the effects of factors such as better co-operation in the taking of medication; following lifestyle modification advice such as losing weight, increasing exercise or stopping smoking; avoiding unnecessary investigations; and carrying out effective post-operative self-care.

It is even more difficult to place a price on patients' peace of mind and mental health when they have a fuller understanding of their health problems and how to deal with them. Yet these are precisely the sort of areas where a nurse practitioner consultation is likely to be more beneficial. Simple comparisons with medicine involving cost per patient completely miss the point of a nurse practitioner service. If anything is to be compared it should be value for money, in the broadest sense, rather than cost per patient seen.

Consumer quality

Asking the patients what they thought of the service is an obvious thing to do. Questionnaires assessing patient satisfaction tend to produce results showing extremely high levels of satisfaction, whatever service is being evaluated. This suggests that they lack discrimination and perhaps alternative approaches might be considered. A post-treatment telephone survey carried out by a neutral third party might produce better quality data than a tick box questionnaire. The telephone approach also allows the researcher to ask further questions about what in particular the patient liked/disliked and why. This sort of data is very difficult to capture on a conventional questionnaire. Consent to telephone needs to be gained at the time of the consultation, however, and the person making the calls has to be an experienced researcher in order to avoid introducing bias into the data.

Quality from the patient's perspective is often measured in terms of patient satisfaction surveys, and these have been used in several studies of nurse practitioner effectiveness (Stilwell *et al.*, 1987; Marsh and Dawes, 1995; Poulton, 1995; Reveley, 1998). At this juncture, therefore, we will give a brief overview of some of the work that has been done on patient satisfaction with health services.

Patient satisfaction

In the foreword to a Royal College of Physicians publication, Leslie Turnbull stated that 'patient satisfaction … is an outcome of health care and, like any other outcome, requires measurement' (Fitzpatrick and

Hopkins, 1993). Thus any change to the service offered to patients must be evaluated from the patient's perspective. Fawcett-Henesy (1991) argues that research is needed to find out which patients are willing to use a nurse practitioner and why.

Assessment of patient satisfaction as a quality assurance measure is not unproblematic, however. Vuori (1991), for example, states that we do not know whether the measurement of patient satisfaction has improved the quality of care. He argues that the problem with general assessments of satisfaction is that 'they do not give enough clues for corrections'. Patients may have varying levels of satisfaction with different aspects of care, and this may not come to light. Moreover, opinions of friends and relatives or the patient's own attitudes to health can affect perceptions of satisfaction. Patients' satisfaction with care also depends on the expectations about the care they will receive, which are subjective and are affected by educational, psychological, cultural and experiential factors. Vuori lists several arguments that have been put forward to 'oppose or belittle the role of patient satisfaction':

- Patients lack the scientific and technical knowledge to assess the quality of care
- Patients' physical or mental states may impede objective judgements
- The rapid pace of events – nursing, diagnostics, treatment – prevents patients from having a comprehensive and objective view of care
- Physicians and patients may have different goals; the physicians may even find the patients' wishes harmful or not in their best interests
- Patient satisfaction cannot be measured in a way that yields useful results because it is difficult to define what 'quality' means to patients
- Patients are often reluctant to disclose what they really think because of their sense of dependency on, or prior failures of, patient–physician communication
- Patients cannot accurately recall care process
- Patient surveys or interviews cannot measure subjective phenomena.

Vuori suggests that patient satisfaction surveys usually demonstrate very high levels of satisfaction, often over 90 per cent. The very success of patient satisfaction studies contributes to their dismissal, because it may be seen that 'a phenomenon with so little variation is not worth studying' and 'such results show that there is not a problem worth studying'. Baker suggests that it is not surprising that, in surveys, over 90 per cent of patients report a high degree of satisfaction with a service, because 'the language of satisfaction is too restricted to convey the many nuances of attitude'. Baker (1993, p. 58) suggests that:

... satisfaction is an attitude that follows a process of judgement or cogitation on experiences of the service. Previously held opinions and expectations may influence the judgement. ... Satisfaction is first of all a summary. It is a brief description of so wide a range of experience and belief that it can hardly ever be other than simple acquiescence. ...

Baker argues that if patients are asked if they are satisfied they will say yes – but! It is the 'buts' that need investigation.

If patients are, and should be, partners in their own care, their views must not be invalidated. The rise in the consumer movement, the *Patient's Charter* and market forces have served to transform health care so that it is becoming a 'buyer's market', and this has changed attitudes towards the role of patient satisfaction in quality assurance. Vuori states that 'the goal of quality assurance is no longer technical and professional excellence but optimal quality that meets the needs of patients'. Patient satisfaction measurement enables patients to air their views and gives them the sense of being involved in their own health care. That being so, it is natural to consult patients.

What then is the best way to measure patient satisfaction with regard to the introduction of a nurse practitioner? The most obvious way to elicit responses regarding patients' satisfaction is of course to ask them, but this is not as easy as it seems. McIver (1991) reminds us that asking questions might give us accurate information, but may not necessarily give us information that is useful. Usefulness is related to the purpose to which information is put; we may collect accurate information that has no direct implications for service provision – very interesting, but? Leavey and Wilson (1993) suggest that FHSAs (now health authorities) have been encouraged to use consumer surveys, but without much guidance as to the purpose for which they would be useful. McIver (1991, p. 8) argues that:

Whether the feedback from users will be useful or not is directly connected to the issue of organisational change. If information is collected which will help to improve service quality from the users' perspective, there must be a willingness amongst all staff to change from an organisation which historically 'knows best' what its users need, to one in which users can participate in decisions about their care.

If we want to find out about patients' views on the service provided by the nurse practitioner, we must be able and willing to use that information to improve the service. This is part of the development of a 'patient-oriented service', which Harris (1978; cited in McIver, 1991, p. 9) defines as:

The extent to which the health care organisation is aware of, has concern for, and is responsive to the patient as a 'whole' person ... such a view implies knowledge and behaviour on the part of the organisational staff member appropriate for meeting patients' needs.

Research by Stilwell *et al.* (1987) and Salisbury and Tettersell (1988) shows that nurse practitioners have the knowledge and behaviour to meet patients' needs, and that they treat the patient as a 'whole' person. Stilwell (1987) observed the work of 11 nurses during 339 consultations in the general practice setting. Her study showed support from both patients and doctors for the nurse practitioner role. However, the effectiveness of the role in terms of patient outcomes or alternative professional roles was not addressed. Patients in the evaluation study undertaken by Touche Ross for South Thames Regional Health Authority (Touche Ross, 1994) were found to be highly satisfied with the care which nurse practitioners provided; their consultations were rated in the highest satisfaction category more often compared with those of a group of GP and senior house officer patients. The researchers found that 'nurse practitioner and practice nurse patients were most likely to report the highest levels of satisfaction, between 83% and 84% (excluding non-respondents)' (Touche Ross, 1994). Poulton (1995) also found a high level of patient satisfaction in her small-scale survey of 100 patients in a practice in Yorkshire. However, this practice was atypical in that the practice

population consisted of armed forces personnel and their families, which meant that they were young and highly geographically mobile. Furthermore, the nurse practitioner worked with patients suffering from some form of chronic disease rather than the undifferentiated, acute conditions that many nurse practitioners deal with.

The above studies utilized questionnaires to elicit patient satisfaction with the service. Leavey and Wilson highlight the fact that interactions between users and providers are complex, and can be concerned with a range of issues – for example, accessibility and availability, technical quality, communication, and follow-up. Thus they suggest (Leavey and Wilson, 1993, p. 44):

a single 'blanket' questionnaire covering all aspects wastes effort collecting data on aspects about which there is at present little or no concern, or gathers only superficial data about aspects that are a current concern.

In evaluating patient satisfaction with the nurse practitioner service, availability, communication, technical skill and follow-up are eminently suitable areas for research. But which patients do we ask, and how do we do the asking? Richardson and Maynard (1995) argue that much of the research on nurse practitioner effectiveness fails to measure intermediate and long-term outcomes for patients. Outcome evaluation can be done by examining activity data since the introduction of the nurse practitioner and comparing it with data before he or she was employed. This can in no way demonstrate a straightforward cause and effect relationship, however, as too many variables change over time. Longer term evaluation can only take place over several years, and these studies are very expensive. Furthermore, they assume that the same nurse practitioner will remain in post until the end of the study period.

We have suggested above that both quantitative and qualitative data are required in order to investigate thoroughly all the effectiveness or otherwise of nurse practitioner services. Below is a useful model that encompasses both these types of data. Though this model has been in existence for many years, it still has a lot to offer and has been used by Reveley (1997) in her research into nurse practitioners in general practice.

An evaluation model

A useful framework for the collection and analysis of both qualitative and quantitative data is the structure, process and outcome model (Donabedian, 1966). This model is adapted to the case study as follows.

Structure

Under this heading consideration is given to:

- The physical resources available to the nurse practitioner. This is important because function may follow form – e.g. using a consultation room rather than a treatment room, and not wearing a uniform, was found by Stilwell *et al.* (1987) to result in more consultations for advice on personal and emotional problems.
- The length of each consultation. Stilwell *et al.* (1987) found that the length of the consultation affected the content. This seems self-evident, but nevertheless can impact on patient satisfaction and the job satisfaction of the nurse practitioner. It also determines how many people can be seen per session, and this has an impact on the cost effectiveness of the role.
- The structure of relationships between health professionals in the team, skill mix, composition and size of the team.
- Management systems and policies.
- The legal status of the nurse practitioner and insurance cover for this extended role, which is linked to clinical supervision.

Process

This includes how the role is implemented, and why it is successful or unsuccessful. Consideration is given to:

- The development of protocols or guidelines for practice.
- How the learning needs of the nurse practitioner are identified and met.
- Personal and professional development of the nurse practitioner (inter-personal skills and personal effectiveness, e.g. decision making, confidence, skills acquisition).
- Channels of communication between the nurse practitioner and GP, and between the nurse practitioner and other nursing staff.

- The extent of consensus among the team as to what constitutes the role of the nurse practitioner.
- If there are any disparities, what are they, and what consequences do they have for the smooth implementation of the innovation? How will the consequences be dealt with? How can consensus and co-ordination be brought about with the minimum amount of disruption?
- Comparison of patterns of consultation and content of consultations between doctors and nurse practitioner.
- The types of patient/condition the nurse practitioner will be expected to manage on his or her own responsibility.
- Referral patterns – i.e. direct referral to consultants; requests for tests such as pathology, X-rays.
- Prescribing patterns; protocols.

Outcome

This refers to measurable differences in such things as:

- Patterns of consultation rates, comparison of consultations to doctors and nurse practitioner.
- Effect on waiting lists or cancelled operations.
- Effect on junior doctors' workload.
- Patient/client satisfaction – nature of any complaints or positive comments made by patients and/or their relatives.
- Improvement in nurse practitioner's skills – assessment of competencies.
- Effective use of resources – has there been more use made of certain equipment? Has extra equipment been required? Has staff time been saved? Whose, and by how much? When?
- Effects on skill mix – has there been any reallocation of tasks and responsibilities among staff arising from the introduction of a nurse practitioner?
- Improvements in collaboration between team members.
- Kinds of feedback, if any, received from other agencies involved in patient care.
- Evidence of any illness, etc., going unnoticed, or any incidence of misdiagnosis or errors of treatment/management.

The suggestions outlined above are just some of the ways in which the role of the nurse practitioner can be evaluated. There are many ways of tackling evaluation. Evaluation of the success of the nurse practitioner initiative based on the premise espoused by Fox (1993) would suggest that there is no single resolution of a problem; what counts as a good outcome is often disputed – a number of possible solutions suggest themselves depending on one's position. Fox (1993, p. 742) argues that we need to:

... reject rationality as the keystone to evaluation. Instead, we should acknowledge the presence of a variety of rationalities, each reflecting not Truth, but versions of reality constituted via interests. Evaluation can at least expose those interests if not disclose the path to reason ... postmodernism fragments, it offers new possibilities for action.

A post-modern explanation of the nurse practitioner role would accept the fact that the role can be structured and enacted and its success assessed in different ways at one and the same time.

Conclusion

This chapter has stressed that both quantitative and qualitative approaches to research have their place in evaluating nurse practitioner services. The multidisciplinary nature of nurse practitioner projects should always be considered in designing such a study. A common aim is to investigate how the nurse practitioner service compares with existing services, and either an RCT or time series design is probably the best approach to follow in terms of gathering objective data. The RCT is accepted in medical circles as providing the strongest evidence, but for logistical reasons there are situations where a time series design will have to be used. There are other situations, however, where a largely qualitative approach is needed, as a quantitative methodology is inappropriate. This could be because the research question is to find out how the service impacts upon the users, or because the nature of the client group involved may make an RCT impossible. Whatever the project, it is essential to involve local university staff to ensure academic rigour in the research process. Clear statements of the project goals are essential if the researchers are to be able to ask the right questions and gather the correct data. The three dimensions of professional, managerial and consumer quality should always be considered in designing an evaluation strategy.

We have also suggested that when introducing such a radical new role into the health care team, a simple linear model of evaluation is of limited value. So many factors are involved in the introduction of a nurse practitioner that a wide perspective is required. The work of Smith and Cantley (1985) and Beattie (1984) has done much to illuminate the complex world of evaluation research. At the end of the day the questions to be asked are: Are nurse practitioners successful? And if so, in what ways?

Nurse practitioner services remain fundamentally about nursing, and therefore evaluation of such services should be nurse led. Careful and rigorous application of research principles may be time consuming, but will produce a better service in the long run. This chapter was introduced with a quotation about apple blossom, and it is fitting to end it with a reminder that apple blossom, however attractive it may look, is only transient. What really matters is the care and attention the apple tree receives, as this will ensure its health and vigour. Research and evaluation of nurse practitioner services are therefore very important, as building up a strong evidence base for practice will ensure the health and vigour of the nurse practitioner concept in the long term.

References

Baker, R. (1993). Use of psychometrics to develop a measure of patient satisfaction for general practice. In: *Measurement of Patients' Satisfaction with Their Care* (R. Fitzpatrick and A. Hopkins, eds), p. 58. Royal College of Physicians.

Beattie, A. (1984). *Evaluating Community Health Initiatives: an Overview Paper for NCVO/LVSC Conference. Community Development in Health: Addressing the Confusions.* King's Fund Centre.

Bulmer, M. (1982). *The Uses of Social Research: Social Investigation in Public Policy Making.* George Allen & Unwin.

Carley, M. (1982). *Rational Techniques in Policy Analysis.* Heinemann.

Department of Health (1996). *Promoting Clinical Effectiveness; A Framework for Action in and Through the NHS.* HMSO.

Donabedian, A. (1966). Evaluating the quality of medical care. *Millbank Memorial Fund Q. Bull.*, **44**, 166–203.

Dowling, S., Martin, R., Skidmore, P. *et al.* (1996). Nurses taking on junior doctors' work: a confusion of acccountability. *Br. Med. J.*, **312**, 1211–14.

Fawcett-Henesy, A. (1991). The British scene. In: *Nurse Practitioners: Working for Change in Primary Health Care Nursing* (J. Salvage, ed.). King's Fund Centre.

Fitzpatrick, R. and Hopkins, A. (eds) (1993). *Measurement of Patients' Satisfaction with Their Care.* Royal College of Physicians.

Fox, N. (1993). *Postmodernism, Sociology and Health*, p. 742. Open University Press.

Goldberg, E. M. and Connelly, N. (1982). *The Effectiveness of Social Care for the Elderly.* Heinemann.

Hunter, P. (2000) A woman-centred multi-agency approach to a nurse practitioner-led drop-in centre for prostitutes in Belfast. Eighth International Nurse Practitioner Conference, Abstract, San Diego, September.

Illsley, R. (1980). *Professional or Public Health?* Nuffield Provincial Hospitals Trust.

Leavey, R. and Wilson, A. (1993). Developing instruments for the measurement of patient satisfaction for family health service authorities. In: *Measurement of Patients' Satisfaction with Their Care* (R. Fitzpatrick and A. Hopkins, eds), p. 44. Royal College of Physicians.

MacNeice, L. (1982). Apple blossom. In: *The Rattle Bag* (S. Heaney and E. Hughes, eds). Faber and Faber.

Marsh, G. N. and Dawes, M. L. (1995). Establishing a minor illness nurse in a busy general practice. *Br. Med. J.*, **310**, 778–80.

McIver, S. (1991). *Obtaining the Views of Users of Health Services.* King's Fund Centre.

Øvetreit, J. (1992). *Health Service Quality.* Blackwell.

Polit, D. and Hungler, B. (1995). *Nursing Research; Principles and Methods*, 5th edn. J. B. Lippincott.

Poulton, B. (1995). Keeping the customer satisfied. *Primary Health*, **5(4)**, 16–19.

Reveley, S. (1997). *Introducing a Nurse Practitioner into General Medical Practice; The Maryport Experience.* A report prepared for North Cumbria Health Authority in Association with University College of St Martin, Carlisle.

Reveley, S. (1998). The role of the triage nurse practitioner in general medical practice: an analysis of the role. *J. Adv. Nursing*, **28(3)**, 584–91.

Reveley, S. (1999). Introducing the nurse practitioner into a group general medical practice: operational and theoretical perspectives on role. Unpublished PhD thesis, University of Lancaster.

Richardson, G. and Maynard, A. (1995). *Fewer Doctors? More Nurses? A Review of the Knowledge Base of Doctor–Nurse Substitution.* Discussion Paper 135, York Centre for Health Economics, York Health Economics Consortium, NHS Centre for Reviews and Dissemination.

Sakr, M., Angus, J., Perrin, J. *et al.* (1999). Care of minor injuries by nurse practitioners or junior doctors: a randomised controlled trial. *Lancet*, **354**, 1321–6.

Salisbury, C. J. and Tettersell, M. (1988). Comparison of the work of a nurse practitioner with that of a general practitioner. *J. R. Coll. GPs*, **38**, 314–16.

Smith, G. and Cantley, C. (1985). *Assessing Health Care: A Study in Organisational Evaluation.* Open University Press.

Smith, G. and May, D. (1980). The artificial debate between rationalist and incrementalist models of decision making. *Policy Politics*, **8(2)**, 147–61.

Stilwell, B., Greenfield, S., Drury, V. W. M. and Hull, F. M. (1987). A nurse practitioner in general practice: working style and pattern of consultations. *J. R. Coll. GPs*, **37**, 154–7.

Sutherland, D. (1951). *Gertrude Stein: A Biography of her Work.*

Touche Ross (1994). *Evaluation of Nurse Practitioner Projects.* Touche Ross Management Consultants Ltd.

Vuori, H. (1991). Patient satisfaction – does it matter? *Quality Assurance Health Care*, **3(3)**, 183–9.

World Health Organisation (1981). *Health Programme Evaluation: Guiding Principles*, p. 9. WHO.

12
CONCLUSIONS

Shirley Reveley, Mike Walsh and Alison Crumbie

The flag of morn in conqueror's state
Enters at the English Gate:
The vanquished eve, as night prevails,
Bleeds upon the road to Wales.

From *The Welsh Marches*
by A. E. Housman (1896)

So wrote Housman about sunrise and sunset over Shrewsbury in his classic poem telling the story of the border wars between the English and Welsh over many centuries. There are times when nurse practitioners feel they are caught up in a similar struggle in the 'Medical Marches' of today's National Health Service. In years to come it is hoped that people will look back and wonder what all the fuss was about, as the nurse practitioner has become another valuable member of the health care team. By then we hope it will have become accepted that the nurse practitioner is not a nurse practising medicine, but rather a nurse delivering health care in new and innovative ways.

Discussion of the nurse practitioner role will go nowhere if all we have are sterile debates about the meaning of terms such as 'specialist', 'advanced', 'clinical specialist', 'advanced practitioner', etc., as this means little to the patient. Medieval theology spent centuries wrapped in such arcane debates, arguing for example how many angels could dance upon the head of a pin. Such debates achieved nothing but the imprisonment of Galileo and the holding back of our whole modern understanding of the world. Twenty-first century health care needs put the needs of the patient first and foremost, and spend less time pandering to professional egos and the rigid thinking of self-important bureaucrats! Once we concentrate on delivering the best health care possible to patients regardless of the professional tribe to which we belong, the nurse practitioner will be seen as indispensable. The unique combination of medical skills within a nursing context that the nurse practitioner

brings to the patient has transformed care already, and the more this approach is rolled out across the NHS (and the private sector) the bigger the impact will be. The traditionally dominant position of medicine is slowly having to give way as a combination of patient needs, manpower and resource factors and the potential of the nurse practitioner to meet those needs is being recognized. As Thomas Nashe observed in 1590, even 'Swords may not fight with fate' – and neither can medicine.

This book celebrates the role of the nurse practitioner, especially in a hospital setting. It is to a large degree written by and is edited by three proponents of the role who are heavily involved in promoting the role and educating nurses to undertake it. All three of us have been involved, in one way or another, in evaluating the role over a number of years, so are aware of the criticisms levelled at nurse practitioners, and of the culture shift that has been required within the social organization of health care to enable the role to become part of the mainstream of health care delivery. We argue against the role of the nurse practitioner as simply a substitute for medicine; we see it as just another way of delivering good-quality health care. We are convinced that, with the right kind of education and support, the nurse practitioner role is safe and effective, and research certainly shows that patients are in favour of it.

Throughout the book we have drawn on a wealth of research and commentary about the role, and the following sections summarize the main implications of the nurse practitioner role in British health care at the current time.

The nurse practitioner as doctor substitute

Richardson and Maynard (1995) state that the results of studies suggest that between 30 and

70 per cent of doctors' tasks could be carried out by nurses, although they warn us that many of the studies suffer from a lack of external validity. It has been suggested elsewhere (Reveley, 1999) that Richardson and Maynard's stance on nurse practitioners is too narrow a view of the role; the nurse practitioners do take on some tasks previously located within the domain of medical practice, but they also bring a nursing focus to the consultation that patients value. However, the increasing interchangeability between nurse and doctor does signal a reduced reliance on doctors, and this has implications for the division of labour in a cost-conscious policy era. If nurse practitioners extend their role into the medical domain, is this because the interests of patients will be better served, because it will facilitate the professionalization of nursing, or because it will help answer a crisis in medicine brought about by the New Deal for junior doctors? Perhaps all of these factors interrelate, and the proponents of the nurse practitioner role have seen the opportunities afforded by the National Health Service reforms to carve out a niche for themselves.

As nurses become more involved in nurse-led interventions such as assessment clinics and chronic disease management, it is uneconomic and inefficient to refer to medical colleagues those aspects of clinical care that can be managed well by appropriately educated nurses. As Walsh argued in Chapter 2, the issue of power and vested interests is central to the debate on nurse practitioners. The boundaries between medicine and nursing, though blurring, are fraught with medico-legal pitfalls that need to be urgently addressed. Government White Papers and reports urge interprofessional collaboration and interdisciplinary teamworking, yet until nurses have a strong voice and the knowledge and political awareness to be advocates for themselves as well as patients the profession's subservience to medicine will continue.

The fact that the introduction of the nurse practitioner role has served to blur the boundaries between medicine and nursing has important implications for role boundaries, and marks a major shift in health care provision. Oberschall (1974; cited in Maurin, 1980) suggests that 'conditions which favour challenge to an institutionalized order are those which signal relaxation of social control so that the risk/reward ratio changes for some group'. The risk/reward ratio related to nurse practitioners has changed. Extensive research in the USA and UK (for example, Touche Ross, 1974; Coopers and Lybrand, 1996) has demonstrated that nurse practitioners are safe and effective, and are appreciated by patients. The problems of recruitment into general practice and the reduction in junior doctors' hours has meant that increasing numbers of the medical profession are finding the nurse practitioner role acceptable. Importantly, *The Scope of Professional Practice* (UKCC, 1992) has provided a framework for extending nursing roles. These structural factors provide the 'space' (Svensson, 1996) for nurse practitioners to negotiate around the rules of medical and nursing practice.

Nurse practitioners and nursing

This of course has implications for nursing itself. Does the introduction of the nurse practitioner role recreate two tiers in nursing? Memories of the RGN/EN divide are still fresh for many nurses. Will nurse practitioners undertake the tasks that are perceived by some as 'elite', as they are tasks that doctors formerly carried out? This will leave other nurses with the routine nursing work, and perhaps the development of the health care assistant, recently granted membership of the Royal College of Nursing, could lead to a third tier of nursing. Some would argue that this is the case, particularly when the nurse practitioner role is often linked to education at degree level. Furthermore, the UKCC has been very reluctant to protect the nurse practitioner title by making it a recordable qualification, so that at present any nurse in the UK can call him- or herself a nurse practitioner and claim increased levels of autonomy in practice.

How does the expanded nurse practitioner role that relieves doctors of some of the burdens of routine work affect the autonomy of nurses? Walby and Greenwell (1994) suggested that '... in-so-far as a market has been introduced into the NHS it is not between producer and consumer but between producers'. The market they referred to has, of course, disappeared with the Conservative government that set up the internal market.

However, the importance of value for money and effective use of scarce resources rightfully remains. It may be argued that hospital consultants have more power in terms of managerial responsibility and control of resources, and this may result in limited extension of the nursing role, but only on medical terms. This will reduce the autonomy of nurses to engage in nursing. If nurse practitioners extend their role by simply taking on the tasks delegated to them by doctors, they will require close supervision from doctors. Apart from reducing their autonomy, this would leave nurses in a position of responsibility without authority – a situation that makes nurses vulnerable to the vagaries of a more powerful profession. The extended role of the nurse will be acceptable to managers and doctors, as it increases patient flow, reduces the pressure on doctors and maintains the hierarchical relationship between doctors and nurses. Furthermore, if the promised expansion of recruitment into medical school takes place, then a few years from now, as more newly qualified doctors appear on the scene looking for jobs, those nurse practitioners who are effectively temporary 'medical stopgaps' will become redundant. Current medical shortages have created opportunities for nurse practitioners but, as the above argument demonstrates, it would be folly to define the nurse practitioner role purely in terms of a medical substitute.

On the other hand, nurses could expand their role by entering into partnerships with patients and doctors, having responsibility for a case load, admitting patients to and discharging them from the health care system, referring to other agencies including consultants, and becoming involved in teaching junior doctors about health care. As this chapter is being written, the Department of Health is consulting about prescriptive authority for nurses. At least two of the five options being presented represent a dramatic expansion in nursing roles, as they would give appropriately trained nurses the authority to prescribe a wide range of medicines. Nurses would have to adhere closely to the UKCC (1992) *Scope of Professional Practice* guidelines, however, to prescribe safely, and of course accept close scrutiny and audit of their practice. This expanded and much more autonomous role can be seen as more of a threat to both medicine and general management because it allows for the nurse–patient partnership to become an alternative to the patient–doctor partnership (Witz, 1994). It does however, give the potential for a new nurse–doctor partnership to emerge on an equal footing, which could evolve ideally into a patient–nurse–doctor triad. The extended role as defined above is familiar and more acceptable to doctors as it means relieving them of routine tasks, especially if these have been undertaken by junior doctors (Witz, 1994). However, the expanded role has much more to offer patients and need not threaten medicine. It is about health care delivery, not about nurses practising medicine.

It could be argued that medicine is very slowly undergoing a process of proletarianization whilst nursing is undergoing a process of professionalization, resisting the handmaiden image and seeking more egalitarian ways of working with doctors. However, extended nursing roles means delegation of tasks from doctors, which bestows responsibility and discretion on nurses but not true autonomy. In this sense nurses could be said to be supporting doctors, and in this situation the professionalization project of nursing would be held back. For nursing to be more autonomous means expanding the nursing role and entering into a true partnership with patients in their own right. This is what many nurse practitioners are attempting to do and why they are met with resistance from both medicine and nursing, for nursing is divided amongst its ranks as to the value of the professionalization project and of nurse practitioners.

Sometimes the profession of nursing appears to be its own worst enemy – for example, in arguing over the issue of whether or not nurse practitioners are merely doctor substitutes. If internal disharmony is allowed to prevail, nurse practitioners will remain marginal to both nursing and medicine and may align themselves to doctors in their own interests. Moreover, in the current changing health service whereby primary care Trusts will be commissioning services for local populations from hospitals, there may be differences in the development of nursing roles throughout the country, depending on the type and quantity of nursing services required in a particular location. It might well be that the core skills of the nurse practitioner are seen as an essential requirement for all nurses working in high-level, autonomous roles. Nurses from all specialities therefore need to come together to really sort out what the nurse of the future will look like before someone else decides this for them. We recommend that a good starting point for such a debate would be the nurse practitioner role.

However, for nurses to come together requires professional confidence. Historically, nursing's subservience to medicine has become institutionalized so that nurses have internal-ized the characteristics of an oppressed group (Roberts, 1996). This oppression, it has been argued, arises from the patriarchal nature of women in society reflected in the doctor–nurse relationship (Gamarnikow, 1978), which allowed doctors historically to control nursing education and practice and created gendered strategies of closure (Witz, 1988, 1994). Because nursing was defined as women's work by nurse reformers of the nineteenth century, and in Nightingale's view being a good nurse was to be first and foremost a good woman, 'the occupational ideology of nursing gen-derised the division of labour' (Robinson, 1991). Changes are required at societal level if established professional and gender power hierarchies within the formal health care system are to be changed (Pizurki *et al.*, 1987). These changes include valuing caring and valuing women, and for nursing to be seen as a responsible, autonomous profession equal in status to other professions. This requires increased status for women in society and a redistribution in the exercise of power between men and women. It means that the work women and nurses do in terms of attending to the physical and emotional needs of people must be acknowledged as vital and not dismissed in terms of 'trivia' or 'support' (Davies, 1995, pp. 60–61). Davies suggests that nursing is, in terms of the above, not a profession but an adjunct to a gendered concept of a profession:

Nursing is the activity, in other words, that enables medicine to present itself as masculine/rational and to gain the power and the privilege of so doing.

Davies goes on to say that nursing has not had the first bite of the cherry in defining its own work, and that what nursing is doing is 'putting a conceptual frame around just those aspects of the work of health and healing that are left over after medicine has imposed an essentially masculinist vision' (Davies, 1995). This is rather a pessimistic view of nursing's quest for professional recognition, but it does get to the heart of the matter.

The current policy framework

There has been an increasing emphasis on teamwork and integration over the past decade, with a need to work within govern-ment guidelines and policies, such as generic prescribing and the GP (General Practitioner) Contract (DoH and the Welsh Office, 1989), and the reduction in junior doctors' hours. These policies have increased the opportuni-ties for nurses to enskill themselves. As a result, there has been a certain amount of skill review and skill-mixing within hospitals that has made some workers more flexible and has provided some nurses with specialist skills. The enskilling of nurses, however, whilst helping to reduce stress among doctors and helping achieve government targets, does not come without a cost. The training elements need to be considered, as does the stress placed on nursing staff by the increased responsibility they are being asked to take on.

The focus on consumer involvement has meant a much greater need to include patients and carers in all aspects of health care delivery, and this has an effect on power relationships between patients, carers and health pro-fessionals at all levels of the service. Beattie (1995) has suggested that we are moving toward 'a new republic of health' by redrawing professional boundaries in health care. What would a republic of health look like? It would involve power sharing among professional groups, and groups would come together functionally to address a problem on more or less equal terms. It is not monarchist, in that one person would not hold power, and it celebrates the contribution of patients and clients as well as professionals.

An optimistic view is that this process is already happening with the advent of primary care Trusts, which is bound to have an effect on the culture of the hospital. The pessimistic view is that this will not happen, as doctors will not be willing to power share. The flexible delivery of health care in the current policy framework includes teamwork, flexibility of roles, integrated teams, and the desire for cost effectiveness. It is becoming apparent that the hospital is developing some features of the 'flexible firm', with the nurse practitioner role being potentially one of flexible specialization. The traditional view of the hospital is that of a bureaucratic organization marked by hierarchical levels of responsibility.

The changing face of health care delivery, with the current emphasis on decentralization, plurality of provision and flexible response to local need, has much in common with postmodernist perspectives on organization. Placing the hospital in the context of postmodernist perspectives on organization helps to explain some of the tensions and contradictions that staff experience. An example of this is the increasing flexibility of the nursing workforce wherein nurses are being encouraged to view themselves as autonomous professionals accountable for their own actions and being responsive to patient need. However, at the same time they are expected to work to protocols as part of a multidisciplinary health care team and to be answerable to managers. One of the dangers of flexibility of the workforce, though, is that it may result in a highly qualified core of workers who have security of tenure, supported by a peripheral labour force of less well qualified workers who are drawn into the workforce as and when necessary. Nurses unable to commit themselves fully to the professional ethos of putting work first may become peripheral workers, with all that implies for the professionalization of nursing. Such workers often find it difficult to access education, for example, and are not always included in decision making and strategic planning within the organization.

Education

That the role (or title) of 'nurse practitioner' is becoming increasingly popular is clear, and the nursing profession must ask why this is occurring and why existing roles such as the clinical nurse specialist role and the community specialist nursing roles are not answering the needs of nurses. It may be that courses of preparation for such nursing roles do not adequately prepare nurses to meet the health care needs of patients as well as they might. For example, professional rhetoric espouses holistic care, yet the fact that nurses cannot prescribe medication, perform a physical assessment, take a complete history and manage straightforward illness flies in the face of holism. Nurse practitioners need to undergo a formal course of education which teaches them to be politically and professionally aware and clinically competent, develops their interpersonal skills and enables them to attain the confidence to express their views and needs. All this, together with the additional skills of assessment and diagnosis, make nurse practitioners eminently marketable as members of the health care team, although not as a cheap alternative to doctors. There is a need for Education Consortia to address the education and training of nurse practitioners in the same way as other nurses. This has implications for protected time for teaching and supervision within the clinical setting. If these were formally set up, standards would be easier to maintain and could be a requirement of Consortia (soon to be Confederation) funding.

One thing is certain; education is not cheap, and nurses will only feel their worth has been truly recognized when the NHS is prepared to invest comparable amounts of resources in post-registration nursing education to that which it does in post-graduate medical education. Cheap and cheerful in-house courses of a week or two will not produce a nurse practitioner. Such a complex and advanced role requires education to at least Honours degree level, and hospital Trusts have got to be prepared to invest in nursing at that level to achieve the full benefits of the nurse practitioner concept. Inadequate in-house training programmes of a few days' duration reminds us of Eberhardt's rhetorical question, 'Was man made stupid to see his own stupidity?' (Eberhardt, 1982).

Patients' perceptions of the nurse practitioner

Many studies have shown that patients value nurse practitioners, particularly their interpersonal skills, the time they have available, their educative function and their clinical competence. Nurse practitioners offer effective, holistic care, based on sound knowledge and skills, and are an acceptable alternative to doctors in many instances. Wholesale substitution of doctors by nurse practitioners, however, would probably not be acceptable to patients; doctors are still seen as the ultimate authority on matters medical (Reveley, 1999). The success of the nurse practitioner role can no longer be doubted and nor can the reasons for this success, but there are still serious limitations to the role, not least of which are the medico-legal implications of nurse practitioner practice. The role of the nurse practitioner should be recognized, not in terms of a role that is characterized by doctor-substitution and evaluated in terms of economics and efficiency, but rather as one that encompasses nursing, medical, teaching and health promotion dimensions, and is judged on the basis of what it has to offer in a variety of situations and in response to a variety of patient or client needs. In other words, for its flexibility in the face of an ever-changing health care system. Let us not erect boundaries around the role that serve to strangle its development, but instead allow it to develop in a fluid, dynamic manner. That is not to say that the role must be so elastic that it becomes diffuse and meaningless – we are well aware of the arguments that if nurses are all things to all people they lose their value and their work becomes defined and controlled by others. What we are arguing for is for the nursing profession to take control of the nurse practitioner role and use it flexibly in such a way that nursing is empowered and does not become an occupation that substitutes for other professions that are in trouble.

Because there is no official role definition for nurse practitioners, there can be no official standard of education and practice. The nurse practitioner role must be negotiated in each and every setting where nurse practitioners work, and must be continually reconstituted in the light of the growing body of research on nurse practitioners, the fast pace of change in health care delivery, and increased consumer expectations. The nurse practitioner role must be negotiated on a continuous basis, and negotiation around the 'rules' of what is nursing and what is medicine does take place, especially when new staff enter the setting.

However, nursing does not exist in a vacuum; changes must occur in medicine, at government level and within other health care professions if the structure of relationships within the health care professions is to change. It is obvious that there are objective differences in power that structure relationships within the health care organization, notably the power held by doctors over others in practice. As Freidson (1971) noted: 'A dominant profession stands in an entirely different structural relationship to the division of labour than does a subordinate profession.' The issues involved are bigger than nursing alone; the prospects for nursing are bound up with the whole terrain of interprofessional relationships, statutory bodies and grand policy.

References

Beattie, A. (1995). War and peace among the health tribes. In: *Interprofessional Relations in Health Care* (K. Soothill, L. Mackay and C.Webb, eds), p. 22. Edward Arnold.
Coopers and Lybrand (1996). *Nurse Practitioner Evaluation Project: Final Report*. NHS Executive.
Davies, C. (1995). *Gender and the Professional Predicament of Nursing*, pp. 60–61. Open University Press.
Department of Health and the Welsh Office (1989). *General Practice in the National Health Service: A New Contract*. HMSO.
Eberhardt, R. (1982). The fury of aerial bombardment. In: *The Rattlebag* (S. Heaney and T. Hughes, eds). Faber and Faber.
Freidson, E. (1971). *Professional Dominance*. Atherton.
Gamarnikow, E. (1978). Sexual division of labour: the case of nursing. In: *Feminism and Materialism* (A. Kuhn and A. M. Wolpe, eds). Routledge and Kegan Paul.
Housman, A. E. (1939). The Welsh Marches. In: *The Collected Poems of A. E. Housman*. Penguin.
Maurin, J. (1980). Negotiating an innovative health care service In: *The Sociology of Health Care: Professional Control of Health Services and Challenges to Such Control*, Vol. 1 (J. Roth, ed.). JAI Press Inc.
Nashe, T. (1590). Adieu, Farewell Earth's Bliss. In: *The Rattlebag* (S. Heaney and T. Hughes, eds). Faber and Faber.
Oberschall, A. (1974) *Social Conflict and Social Movements*. Prentice Hall.
Pizurki, H., Jejia, A., Butter, J. and Ewart, L. (eds) (1987). *Women as Providers of Health Care*. World Health Organisation.
Reveley, S. (1999). Introducing the nurse practitioner into a group general medical practice: operational and theoretical perspectives on role. Unpublished PhD thesis, University of Lancaster.

Richardson, G. and Maynard, A. (1995). *Fewer Doctors? More Nurses? A Review of the Knowledge Base of Doctor–Nurse Substitution*. Discussion Paper 135, York Centre for Health Economics, York Health Economics Consortium, NHS Centre for Reviews and Dissemination.

Roberts, S. J. (1996). Breaking the cycle of oppression: lessons for nurse practitioners? Point of view: *J. Am. Acad. NPs*, **8(5)**, 209–13.

Robinson, J. (1991). Power and policy making in nursing. In: *Nurse Practitioners: Working for Change in Primary Health Care Nursing* (J. Salvage, ed.). King's Fund Centre.

Svensson, R. (1996). The interplay between doctors and nurses – a negotiated order perspective. *Sociol. Health Illness*, **18(3)**, 379–98.

Touche Ross (1994). *Evaluation of Nurse Practitioner Projects*. Touche Ross Management Consultants Ltd.

United Kingdom Central Council (1992). *The Scope of Professional Practice*. UKCC.

Walby, S. and Greenwell, J. (eds) (1994). *Medicine and Nursing: Professions in a Changing Health Service*. Sage Publications.

Witz. A. (1988). Patriarchal relations and patterns of sex segregation in the medical division of labour. In: *Gender Segregation at Work* (S. Walby, ed.). Open University Press.

Witz, A. (1994). The challenge of nursing. In: *Challenging Medicine* (J. Gabe, D. Kelleher and G. Williams, eds), p. 36. Routledge.